Breathing Out

Karen Hockney

For Iain, Livvy and Issy, who trod the path with me

Above all, be the heroine of your life, not the victim

Nora Ephron

Chapter One

Cancer Doesn't Happen To Perfect Karen

Actually, it does. And while being fit and healthy won't prevent cancer, it puts you in a good place to fight back.

My nickname is Perfect. I run marathons. I'm size eight. I don't smoke. I don't eat junk food. I don't eat meat. But before you throw this book across the room, my perfect little world fell apart on September 15th 2011 when I heard the words no-one ever wants to hear. 'It's bad news, you've got cancer.' The first thing my friends said was: 'Perfect Karen can't have cancer.' If it could happen to me, what chance did my exercise-avoiding, sugar junkie, cigarette and vodka loving buddies have?

For four weeks officially BC (before cancer) I lived under a cloud waiting for test results after finding the small hard lump in my right breast while lying in bed early one morning a month earlier. We were in Florence on the last day of a glorious three week summer road trip through Italy when I felt the hard mass which suddenly stopped my world in its tracks. I pressed it, it bounced back, hard and rigid and immoveable. It didn't hurt and when I looked at myself naked in the mirror, I saw nothing unusual. My husband Iain and I spent that last day in Florence wandering the streets in a daze, stopping in cafes to drink coffee and wine we didn't want and studiously avoiding the subject in front of our two daughters Liv, then 16, and Issy, 12, who were blissfully unaware that anything had changed.

I booked a mammogram as soon as I got home and as the doctor looked at the images on his screen, he said he didn't like the rough edges around the lump – smooth edges are good, but rough edges not so – so he booked me in for a micro-biopsy the following week. The news that I needed a biopsy was a blow, even though I had been expecting to hear it.

I came out of the radiography unit into the waiting room and Iain looked up expectantly. He could see from my face that I hadn't been given the all clear we'd spent a week longing for.

'What did they say?' he asked, his face lined with worry.

'I need a micro-biopsy next week to investigate further,' I said flatly, as big tears started to roll down his face. He grabbed my hand and squeezed it hard.

'Okay, I'm sure it will come back fine,' he said, giving me a wry smile through his tears. 'And if it doesn't, we will get through this, so don't worry.'

'I don't want to tell the girls until we know for sure,' I added, fighting the urge to scream and cry. 'Why is this happening to me?' I wanted to yell but instead I walked back to the car in silence with Iain, hand in hand.

I returned the following week for the biopsy and waiting for those results to come back was without a doubt the worst 10 days of our lives. The doctor tried to reassure me as I left.

'Let's just make sure it's nothing to worry about', he said with a kind smile but a sixth sense told me that I wasn't going to get the all clear.

I made a pact with myself there and then: if the results came back clear, I would have a further investigation. That's how convinced I was that I had cancer.

In the interim, life carried on as before except it was now nothing like before. Suddenly the word cancer seemed to be all around me. Out at lunch when we raised our glasses and someone said, 'To good health,' it felt like there was an omen hanging in the air. I felt anxious, unable to concentrate, breathless and out of control.

Somehow I managed to get through a long-arranged party we had planned and not burst into tears whenever someone asked innocently: 'How are you?' I spent the afternoon and evening in the kitchen, avoiding any kind of deep or meaningful conversation until a few glasses of Champagne had smoothed the edges and rendered me merry enough to push all thoughts of tests and results to the back of my mind.

Pretending that everything was fine in front of the girls on a daily basis during that interminably long three week period was even harder. Both Iain and I were trying to act normal while the nightmarish thoughts in both our heads dominated every waking hour. I lost my thread in conversations and I stopped moaning about untidy bedrooms and bathroom towels being left on the floor. Getting up each morning and forcing smiles, laughter, jollity and normal behaviour was unbearable.

Four days before diagnosis, I was asked to report on a dazzling party thrown by Mont Blanc and the Grimaldi family in Monte-Carlo by Hello magazine. A limousine came to pick me up and deliver me to what at any other time would be a night to remember. I saw Bryn Terfel sing at the Opera House before rubbing shoulders at the Champagne reception with Jerry Hall, Daryl Hannah and Natalie Imbruglia. I slipped back into gear, interviewing Naomi Watts, Eva Herzigova, Olivia Palermo and her boyfriend Johannes Huebl amongst others before we went into a sumptuous dinner at the Michelin starred Louis XV restaurant in the Hotel de Paris. To the outside world, I looked the same as usual but going round and round in my head that evening was just one thought: 'Have I got cancer?'

The call I had been dreading finally came through three weeks after my first test. My GP called to say he had received my results. Poor guy, he thought the clinic had already passed on the news but instead found himself in the horrific position of being pressured to tell me over the phone that I had a tumour which needed immediate surgery.

'It's bad, it's hormone receptive breast cancer and you need surgery pretty quickly,' is all he would say, clearly flustered at having to give such horrible news over the phone. 'Please can we go into the detail of this tomorrow in person,' he pleaded and I found myself apologising for wanting to know more and asking too many questions.

How bad is bad was the only question going around in my head as I put the phone down and came downstairs. The glass of rosé I had taken upstairs as Dutch courage for his call was promptly tipped down the sink. Iain was in the kitchen supervising the cooking I had left when the call came from my GP. One look at my face told him all he needed to know. He had almost convinced himself it was going to be a false alarm, a harmless cyst, nothing to worry about.

'Let's have supper, we'll talk about it later,' I said, hearing the voices of the girls outside on the terrace as they laid the table.

Watching the girls at supper as they laughed and joked together was surreal, like an out of body experience. How do you tell your kids you have cancer? All my instincts as a mother had been about protecting them from pain and hurt, shielding them from anything bad and making life as productive, happy and stable as possible. Now my bad news was going to unleash the most horrendous pain and suffering imaginable on them and there was absolutely nothing I could do about it. Well, I could choose to keep it from them but given their ages and my complete lack of acting ability, I knew that this wasn't a realistic option.

'Hey mum, you look like you have a story to tell,' they were cackling. 'Come on, spit it out!' Bizarrely, the most important thing on my mind at that moment was getting them to finish their supper before I broke the news. I knew they wouldn't be able to eat anything afterwards.

Watching those two faces change from carefree laughter to streams of tears as I told them I had breast cancer was something I never want to see again. Having surgery, radiotherapy and even the big bad wolf that is chemotherapy doesn't even begin to touch the pain of watching my sassy, witty, funny, brave girls crack and whimper like babies. Nothing will ever be as difficult as that.

After reassuring them that I would tell them everything and that I was going to fight like a demon to get well, Issy went straight to bed, and straight to sleep. Shock had simply knocked the stuffing out of her. Liv took herself off to her room to try and digest it all.

The evening went by in a haze of what ifs….how long had it been there, could I have detected it any earlier, had it spread? We had no answers just yet and not knowing what we were dealing with was the hardest thing of all. The mystery was that I hadn't come across the lump earlier that summer given that I had spent weeks on the beach, rubbing sun lotion on without noticing a thing. Well, I had been more tired than usual, but given the travelling, socialising and working round the clock at the Cannes Film Festival, a bit of fatigue was hardly surprising.

That night, the tears Iain and I had held back earlier in front of the girls poured forth as we lay together in bed, promising each other that no matter how difficult the path ahead, we would get through it somehow. Iain had got through the previous three weeks of waiting hoping and believing that everything would be okay. We were both going through the motions of normal everyday life but the discovery of that small hard mass had changed everything.

Quieter than usual, in the days BC, he would grab my hand as we sat on the sofa with a glass of wine or watching TV and squeeze it gently three times, which has always been our unspoken way to say I love you. We were already close but sharing this burden and not being able to confide in anyone else had brought us even closer. Once we knew I had cancer, his tears came but they were accompanied by a steely determination that nothing was going to beat me.

'You will get through this Kaz, you are a fighter,' he told me as we lay side by side mulling over the hard road that lay ahead. 'You are so strong and fit and positive, this disease has no chance against you.'

My GP came into his surgery half an hour early to meet us the following morning and go through the results: a grade 1 tumour, the lowest grade of cancer, with oestrogen and progesterone receptors that stimulate growth. The first bit of good news.

'So what timescale are we looking at for surgery?' I asked, wondering if I was still going to be able to fit in the jobs in Los Angeles and western France that I had just confirmed. Not just any old jobs either....an interview with Kathy Bates and a feature on riding with the French cavalry horsemen from the prestigious Cadre Noir horse school. He looked at me like I was slightly mental and gave a wry smile before addressing me by my married name to tell me: 'Mrs Kershaw, you need to cancel, you are not going to be getting on a plane anytime soon.'

An hour later I sat discussing surgery with my surgeon Dr Lanvin (yes, it must have been karma to get a surgeon whose name conjures up images of pretty ballet pumps and perfume.) When we walked into his consulting room, I whispered to Iain: 'Oh my God, it's George Clooney!' He was a little shorter but Dr L bore an uncanny resemblance to one of Hollywood's hottest screen heroes. Being treated by ER's Doug Ross was no bad thing. I did wonder whether I had time to fit in a hair appointment and some highlights before being admitted so I could look my best on the slab. As my journalist friend Clare pointed out once she had stopped crying after I broke the news: 'Kazza, only you could get a doctor who is haute couture and looks like Clooney.'

Imagine sitting bolt upright in a dentist's chair, topless with skirt and shoes on, while George Clooney studies your right breast and decides where to make the incisions for surgery. He'd already seen my date of birth and the 44-year-old me braless so we all knew where we were at.

'I know this sounds shallow but can we just talk about afterwards...will I need reconstruction, and how will it look?' I asked him nervously.

'No reconstruction,' said Clooney in his perfect English with just a hint of French accent. 'The tissue will move back into place naturally and the scar will be very neat. And a woman's body and image is very important so you should ask these questions,' he added. 'It will look, how you say it, a little perkier than the other breast afterwards.'

We both laughed and I asked if he could perform a little lift on the other side while he was at it. 'No need, it will all be fine. Don't worry.'

He explained the procedure: A full thoracic scan and blood tests before an operation to remove the tumour, which was estimated at 18mm. The lymph nodes showed clear in my scans, which meant no chemotherapy unless they found evidence of cancerous cells during the operation. In which case there would be another operation to remove the lymph nodes followed by four months of chemotherapy. Oh yes, and five years of Tamoxifen, the anti-oestrogen drug which stops this hormone from encouraging certain types of breast cancer cell growth.

It's fair to say I didn't expect to be facing a health crisis of this magnitude in my early 40s. The only time I'd stayed overnight in hospital was during the births of Liv and Issy. I'd spent my adult life playing tennis, doing yoga, swimming, running and horse-riding. I took up surfing when I hit 40 and ran the first of two London Marathons. My only vices? Sunbathing and a glass of wine or two. Okay, a bottle or two on a particularly fun night out. Or in. But that week in September 2011, I learned that a clean and healthy lifestyle is no guarantee against serious illness. After a lifetime spent avoiding recreational substances and not even taking paracetamol for a headache, I allowed myself a wry smile at the prospect of turning into a legitimate drug user.

And breathe…..Swot up and become as well informed as possible about your type of cancer, the treatment, the drugs and what to expect. It's like being on a rollercoaster blindfolded and every experience is different but a bit of advance information is never a bad thing.

Chapter Two

A Charmed Life

Laughter makes you feel better, it's a proven medical fact. And without a few inappropriate, in-terribly-bad-taste laughs, this whole cancer malarkey would have been unbearable.

Pre-cancer, my life was pretty exciting. I've had a passion for writing since I was tiny and cut my teeth in news reporting before swapping the depressing world of news for the fluffy orbit of showbiz. I spent six months at the Daily Mail before jumping ship to work with Piers Morgan on the Bizarre pop column at The Sun. My freelance career started in the mid-90s, just before the birth of Liv, and those early years were spent juggling celebrity interviews, documentary filming trips and exotic location visits all over the world with motherhood and a permanently buzzing office in North London. They were heady days....one week I'd be at a lunch with Nelson Mandela in Cape Town, the next I'd be listening to on-set gossip in the back of a limo with Desperate Housewives Eva Longoria and Felicity Huffman. On less fluffy days, I might be interviewing street kids living in the sewers of Bogota or meeting orphans in Bangladesh. Iain was working long hours in the City and the pace of life continued unabated when Issy arrived in 1999.

One dreadful rainy June day in 2007, I had an epiphany as I put away the cushions for our new garden furniture that had yet to be sat on as another cloud burst over our garden. Why not move to the South of France, where we already had an apartment, and start afresh with beautiful weather, lovely food and wine and great culture as well as more time to enjoy family life together?

So it was that after so many farewell parties my liver was in danger of collapse, we left Hertfordshire the following summer on the hottest day of the year in a car packed with two stressed cats, a dog, two kids and everything we had forgotten to put in the removal lorry.

We arrived at our new home, a Provencal villa in Bar sur Loup, one of the prettiest villages on the Côte d'Azur, a stone's throw from the glamour of Cannes and just an hour from the Italian border, ahead of schedule at 6am and had to break into the garden with the huge cat crate as the poor devils were about to collapse with heat exhaustion.

The house hadn't been lived in for several years so there was dust and dirt everywhere, windows you couldn't see through and loos which didn't work properly. We found tree roots climbing up the walls in the downstairs bathroom. The removal men arrived in an enormous truck which couldn't get down our black ski run of a drive so Iain had to hire a smaller van in nearby Grasse to transport our furniture from the village to the house. The spiral staircase was a nightmare...the cats refused to go up or down it...and the electric gate gave up the ghost as soon as the removal men left.

But waking up to the spectacular views of mountains and valley right outside our bedroom window and hearing birds sing instead of boy racers taking the nearest corner made it worthwhile, although as the girls grew older, they made it clear they would welcome the odd boy racer, or even boy, in the vicinity.

Life was good, business was steadily building back up to the pre-France highs for both of us and we enjoyed some amazing times in our adopted community, skiing through the winter, hitting the beaches on the Riviera each summer and generally living la dolce vita.

Getting cancer, and in a foreign country too, was not part of the plan. At first, I was intimidated by the idea of being treated in

France because while I could speak perfectly passable French, my grasp of medical terms was not that hot. It was an enormous relief when I found out that Clooney spoke great English, a legacy of having worked in a large hospital in Montreal. His secretary gave me his mobile number and told me to call him if I had any questions, as she didn't speak English and she was concerned that I understood everything. It was reassuring to know that France's record in cancer treatment pretty much outshone the rest of the western world. My medical vocabulary improved by the day thanks to Google translate and I felt completely chuffed the day I managed to fill in an entire health questionnaire without hesitation. There had to be a reason Kylie Minogue chose to have her treatment for breast cancer in Paris when she could have gone anywhere in the world.

Pre-treatment, the toughest part was breaking the news to my close family and friends. It's not a call you ever want to make to the people you love and who love you. The amazing support that came my way was almost overwhelming. And even at the bleakest of times, there was comedy too. My last call in a weekend spent breaking bad news was to my Californian buddy Susie, who impatiently responded to my constant requests to chat with: 'What's up, are you dying or something?' Many conversations that started with tears and devastation ended with hysterical laughter as I relayed the stupid, funny things about being diagnosed with a life-threatening illness. Like love and hate, there's a thin line between laughter and misery.

A school mum I'd met a couple of times on the drop off and pick up contacted me to offer advice, support and cancer books galore. She had battled breast cancer eight years earlier unbeknownst to her children, who were very young at the time. I passed on her kind offer. Reading has always been an escape for me and my consignment of Surf Mama, The Reluctant Fundamentalist, Waterlog and How To Be A Woman was more appealing than how to beat cancer literature.

One of my oldest journalist friends, Sally, put together a cancer care package full of nice things to cheer me up.

'No bad wigs or fluffy slippers,' I told her, 'but vouchers for Selfridges, cashmere pashminas and signed cheques are all fine.'

She had done this for several other poor souls and told me: 'Don't worry Kazza, I don't jinx anyone with my care kits. The others have all survived apart from one, and she knew she was dying before I sent the package.'

She also told me her school mum friend looked amazing all the way through her treatment. Throughout chemotherapy, she would appear at the school gate at home time looking chic and immaculate.

'I looked worse than she did, in my stained trackie pants and old T shirt,' Sally confided. 'I thought she might look a bit rough during her treatment but no, she looked stunning. I bet you will be the same.'

My dog sitter Helen, who was in the same position as me two years earlier, rang me to talk through treatment. Her take was radiotherapy was a breeze while chemotherapy was pretty rough but losing your hair and eyelashes did have an upside, saving a fortune on tints and waxing. Noticing that I looked a bit downcast after this conversation, lovely Liv promised to shave her hair off if I had to lose mine.

An old school friend also rang. She had breast cancer five years earlier and gave me some excellent advice. Look forward, not back, swap wine for Champagne (as it's less acidic) have a little of what you fancy and don't Google cancer, set too much store by other people's well-meaning advice or think too far ahead.

My mum was beside herself with worry in London. All she wanted to do was pop in for a cup of tea and give me a hug. I'd have given anything for her to be able to do that and be by my side but I wanted her to arrive after my operation and see that I was okay and on the way to recovery.

Issy told her section head at school and on the way home in the car she admitted that she cried while she was telling her. The teacher was very kind - her younger sister had been diagnosed with breast cancer a couple of months before me - and they hugged and made a pact to keep each other posted on our progress.

Then it was time to play the cancer card. Prior to my diagnosis, Liv was having trouble with a few friends and teachers at school, nothing too major but enough to upset the sensibilities of a hormonal teenager. I knocked on her bedroom door.

'I'm making some calls,' I told her. 'The one good thing about having a mum with cancer is that no-one will be horrible to you for the next few months. Tell me if you get any texts.'

Within an hour of me breaking the news, she had received a text from one friend, who turned from being tricky into an angel in the blink of an eye. And the teacher she had spent three years hating with a passion was suddenly all over her like a rash, offering a listening ear and telling her she could be a passenger in lessons for a little while if she wanted!

Being unable to plan ahead for work as a result of constant hospital appointments was the downside to all the lovely years I had spent feeling smug about freelance life. Instead of filling my diary with exciting interviews, TV festivals and jollies abroad, I was writing in blood tests, consultations with Clooney and scans. So when Iain sent me a text one morning while I was waiting for tests saying he had just made his first profit of the day I had the perfect response.

'That's excellent,' I texted back. 'Especially now I'm going to be laid up watching daytime television every day for the next two months.' It occurred to me that being 'seriously ill' meant being off the hook for housework, cooking and conjugal rights for several months, no scratch that, five years actually, thank you Tamoxifen. And despite my sudden lack of earning power, it looked like we'd be in pocket after paying my surgery fees because of what I couldn't spend on new bikinis.

A tranquil calm descended on our usually manic noisy household. The girls stopped arguing and started offering me cups of tea and cuddles in bed. I was allowed to sing along with X Factor contestants without being shouted down. They did everything I asked (sometimes through gritted teeth but without complaining). Unloading the dishwasher, walking the dogs, all the jobs they usually moaned about were completed with barely a word of dissent.

Issy showed signs of niceness fatigue after a few days of enforced goodness but as she rightly pointed out: 'It's not my fault this is happening, is it?' When I remonstrated with her over the fact that her room was still like Armageddon after three requests to tidy up, adding that it wasn't possible for me to clean it even if I wanted to, she responded with: 'OMG can you just stop using the hospital as an excuse for EVERYTHING all the time?'

It was hard for all of us suddenly having this major destructive force in our lives. The girls wanted life to carry on as normal. And normal in our house was lots of animated conversation, people flying off the handle occasionally and everyone talking over each other to say their piece, not people tiptoeing around each other on eggshells frightened to say the wrong thing.

Liv told me: 'Mum I am just going to go to school and do what I usually do and pretend this is not happening. That is the only way I can deal with it.'

'That's fine by me,' I told her. 'And by the way, if there is anything you want to know about what's happening, any questions you want to ask, no matter what, just ask me, don't be afraid. I am going to tell you the truth. Always.'

It wouldn't necessarily be the path to follow with very young children but Liv and Issy possessed a maturity beyond their years and I preferred them to ask me questions than hear half-truths or inaccurate information, however well meant, from friends or acquaintances at school.

Iain and I had had three weeks to get our heads around the idea that something serious might be happening, whereas the girls had this awful bomb explode underneath them with no notice whatsoever. It was hardly surprising that the wrong thing might tumble from their mouths occasionally. In fact, it was reassuring when it did, because it meant that they were feeling normal and had forgotten our troubles for a tiny wee while.

And breathe....You will be bombarded with well-meaning advice, phone calls and offers of support. Trust your instincts and do what feels right for you.

Chapter Three

Welcome To Planet Cancer

Finding a lump early can mean the difference between life and death. Getting to know your body, and your breasts, talking to girlfriends about what to look for, even checking yourself while lying down - which is how I found my lump - instead of standing up, are good habits to get into.

There are lots of weird things about cancer. One is that if you are lucky enough to be diagnosed early, as I was, you don't actually feel ill despite the fact that you have a life threatening illness. I felt absolutely fine physically and looked like the same old me, a picture of health still glowing with a golden tan from our summer in Italy. It's the treatment to make you better that takes you to the brink, not the disease itself, in the early stages at least. Emotionally, I felt strong but little things would tip me into the abyss.

One morning I went to have blood tests at the clinic. They had to do eight tests and as the lab technician counted out the little vials with different coloured tops on, I noticed that I had one each of all of her colour codes.

She caught my eye and asked why I needed so many tests. It felt weird to say I had cancer so I left out the C word and told her I was about to have an operation to remove a tumour. She seemed taken aback despite seeing people like me every day of her working life. As I left after the blood samples were taken she called out: 'Bon courage.' I don't know how I didn't start howling. But once I got used to saying the C word out loud, I realised it would come in quite handy. Being able to flutter my eyelashes and flash my scar and puncture marks would certainly make parking a lot easier during tourist season.

The scans of my ovaries, uterus, diaphragm, liver, kidneys and lungs came back clear, which was a huge relief. The French healthcare system is a thing of wonder, putting you in charge of your medical notes, scans and tests results so if you are having trouble dissecting all the information, you can go back over it at your own pace. My large white envelope containing a complete breakdown of all the latest test results had one key phrase, the magic words: 'Conclusion: Actuellement normale.' After 'Je t'aime', they soon became the next best three words in the French language.

Clooney told me I'd need to sleep in a sports bra for a week after the operation. Cue a shopping trip to Decathlon as there was no way he was going to see the tatty grey sports bra I used for tennis and running. I found a pretty white one with hooks at the back, which was fairly crucial as pulling it on over my head would be impossible after the op. Inexplicably, I also bought some sports socks I didn't need. Heading to a sports shop to equip myself for an operation was a first.

A week before the operation, the enormity of what was about to happen began to sink in. I hunted through the shed for the paint spattered tape measure we'd used during years of house renovating and measured out 18 mm. Less than 2 cms, it didn't sound like much but touching the lump, suddenly it felt huge. It had also started to throb occasionally as if to taunt me, 'Hey, look at me! Still here!' I felt like gouging it out with a knife. Lying comfortably on my right side in bed was impossible.

That evening as we sat on the terrace eating supper, I asked the girls if they had any questions. Liv took a deep breath and said: 'What is the worst thing that can happen when you have your operation?'

'Well, if they find cancerous cells when they remove some of my lymph nodes for testing, they will have to remove quite a few more and I will have to have chemotherapy.' She looked relieved that there was no mention of dying on the operating table.

'This time next week, that cancer alien will be in a specimen jar where it belongs,' I added brightly.

'Yay to that,' she, Issy and Iain chorused.

Another Planet Cancer fact: It makes you tired. Really tired. I searched and racked my brains for anything that had changed in my general wellbeing over the preceding few months that might have given some indication that all was not well with my health and this was the big revelation. Those nasty C cells sap your energy as they mutate and grow, leaving you feeling like you are permanently in training for a marathon. I know that feeling, having run London twice, and the lack of energy by the time evening arrived, coupled with the zonking straight to sleep as soon as my head hit the pillow was reminiscent of the long training days only this time, without any of the long runs.

One evening I put on my running gear and took the dogs out for a 15 minute run before supper. It was hardly worth getting changed but having felt so exhausted the previous week that I could have fallen asleep bolt upright, I had a sudden burst of energy and decided to milk it. I had been for a 10 minute swim earlier. Ten minutes! It was nothing to get worked up about but it felt good just doing something.

My desire to keep fit got me into all sorts of trouble in the week preceding the operation. You know that saying it never rains but it pours? Well, chez Kershaw, it positively pisses down. Clooney had prescribed arnica to help reduce the swelling and bruising after surgery but I had to start taking it five days earlier than planned as I had an argument with a fig tree while walking the dogs and ended up with a black eye and a large angry cut on the eye socket. I saw one ripe fig hanging tantalisingly just out of reach, leaned up to grab it and the bough promptly bounced back in my face. I love figs but this one really wasn't worth it.

With five days to go before D Day, I took off for the beach thinking that relaxation, sunshine and swimming in the sea would be calming for the soul as well as good exercise. As I swam my second loop around the beautiful bay at Theoule, near Cannes, I felt the unmistakable sharp pique of a jellyfish stinging my right hip. With my black eye, diseased boob and red raw hip rash, I found myself saying out loud: 'Please God, let that be my three things.' The only upside was the tall, tanned, blonde beach club boss Steve coming over to bathe it with vinegar, which was the best way to remove the sting and make me smile again.

It struck me as I looked around at the other bathers on the beach that there must be other cancer survivors nearby, maybe even sitting next to me, who had battled back to good health and were leading perfectly normal lives. It was an encouraging thought. A guitarist sat on the rocks playing Spanish guitar melodies with a sax player. As they improvised together I couldn't help thinking that despite incurring an extra injury, it was perhaps the most uplifting way to spend an afternoon.

The good feeling continued that evening. I was too tired to go out so I invited a gaggle of girlfriends over for a curry night. There are very few Indian restaurants in the South of France, and some of the very limited Google research into cancer that I had allowed myself mentioned that curry spices, and particularly turmeric, had marvellous cancer fighting properties. The girls arrived laden down with home-made curries and Champagne while I floated around in impossibly high Prada wedges and a silk dress. I figured they'd be seeing a lot of me prone on the sofa in my PJs for weeks to come so an effort had to be made.

As we chinked glasses, I whipped out my boob and made each one of them feel the lump so they knew exactly what to look for when doing breast examinations. There was lots of prodding and squeezing and ooh-ing and ah-ing and once they had all promised to book a mammogram, we left the C word alone. In France, breast screening starts once you hit your late 30s while in the UK, women have to wait until they reach 50. It's a strange conundrum given that hormone receptive breast cancer seems increasingly to affect women in their 40s. As a result of my droning on, a couple of friends in London booked their first mammograms - opting to pay privately rather than wait for NHS screening to start - and while I couldn't say it made my situation worthwhile, it felt like my journey was also going to yield some good things.

As the days sped by and my date with Clooney loomed, I did

whatever I could to take my mind off the operation. Heading off early one Sunday morning for a mile long swim in the bay of Cannes with some girlfriends, I felt invigorated and invincible and do you know what? A little bit normal again. As I drove home enveloped by the most wonderful physical fatigue, I decided to treat cancer as just another project. Perhaps not quite as interesting as the interview I did with Tamara Ecclestone in Saint-Tropez on her mega bucks superyacht in the summer, just a few weeks before my diagnosis, but talk of her £1 million specially sourced crystal bath for her new London home certainly took my mind off the operating table.

And breathe….Swim in the sea as often as you can (even if you need a wet suit.) You will not believe the healing power of a sea swim or paddle.

Chapter Four

On The Slab

You may think you are superwoman. I truly believe I am. But there is a reason why the doctors tell you to take it easy after surgery and it makes sense to listen, no matter how much your inner domestic goddess wants to argue the toss and do it your way. Turning 40 was a watershed for me. Since that milestone birthday, I had run two marathons, moved to the South of France and started writing a blog. Beating cancer was next on my 'Things to do in your 40s' list. Missing a girl's weekend in Aix-en-Provence with my London friends was disappointing but somehow easier to bear when I reminded myself that instead of shopping, lunching and dancing until way too late in Aix's coolest bar, I would be fighting cancer instead. No contest.

September 27th 2011 arrived, Operation Eve, with a battery of tests planned in advance of surgery the next day. I did my weekly yoga class on the terrace at home with my friend Fiona, who lives in our valley, and my yoga teacher Faye, also a neighbor and a friend. Carrying on with our weekly yoga sessions was vitally important to me and a little piece of sanity and serenity in an increasingly insane world. After a particularly enjoyable session, we said emotional farewells, all managing to bite our bottom lips and not cry, and I disappeared off to pack my bag.

Iain drove me to hospital with a little case full of goodies. My nicest underwear, my prettiest pyjamas, Vogue, Grazia, Hello and books galore as well as my laptop, iPad and a stash of DVDs in case I got bored.

I had jabs full of dye injected into my right nipple and an MRI scan marking the three lymph nodes which would be removed during surgery and tested to see if the cancer was localized or already spreading. If these tests were clear, the remaining lymph nodes would be left alone, but if there was further evidence of cancer cells in them, a number of extra lymph nodes would be removed in the course of the operation. Finally, the indelible cross marking the spot on my right boob was made, just above my nipple where the lump was.

The girls came to visit after school armed with sushi to replace the questionable hospital fare that seems common the world over. Any worries they had about seeing me in hospital were quickly replaced by impressed sighs and gasps as they wandered around the immaculate private room I had opted to pay extra for instead of choosing a small communal ward with three other women. I wasn't in the mood to chat or make new friends, I wanted solitude and to be in and out of hospital as quickly as possible.

'Mum, do you get room service here, and do you have a mini fridge in your room?' demanded Issy as she rushed around the private suite overlooking the leafy hospital grounds, snapping pictures excitedly on her mobile phone. 'Oh my God, you even have two sinks, this place is amazing!'

'I doubt it darling, this isn't a hotel you know,' I told her as I tucked into maki rolls, 'although I have stayed in hotels that are not as luxurious as this.' Spotlessly clean, with a spacious bathroom, power shower, plasma TV, Wi-Fi, safe, air conditioning and a sunny private terrace, all that was missing was a sun lounger and a pina colada.

They squeezed onto the bed either side of me, chatting away happily and filling me on their day at school, their test results and various teachers who had been in a bad mood before reluctantly getting up to leave. I cuddled them harder than usual as they kissed my cheeks and wished me luck for the next day, promising to text and phone from school to see how I was. Iain hugged me tight and whispered: 'Sleep tight, this time tomorrow it will all be over.' He did a great job of keeping a lid on his emotions. I could see he was desperately worried but he hid it well as he chivvied the girls out of my room citing homework and the curry he was going to cook them when they got home.

Clooney popped in on his way home to tell me that the operation was scheduled for 8am the next day. It would take an hour or so, I would be left to heal for three to four weeks before starting radiotherapy and I needed to come back a week later to find out the pathology results of the lump and the final conclusive results of the tests on my lymph nodes. Clooney told me he would call Iain's mobile straight after the operation to let him know how it went.

I loaded Bridesmaids onto the iPad and curled up, mentally punching the air at the thought of the nightmare coming to an end and the nasty toxic little alien finally getting its marching orders.

I was wheeled down to theatre at 7.45am the following morning and woke up three hours later in the recovery room feeling like I had an enormous hangover. Clooney came straight in to see me as I came round from the anaesthetic.

'The surgery went well, the good news is we removed three lymph nodes and we found no cancer in any of them.' He squeezed my hand adding: 'Please don't worry anymore.'

'If you're pleased, I'm pleased,' I beamed back at him woozily. Even in my zonked out state, I understood that I had clear lymph nodes and it was the best result I could have wished for.

I spent the rest of the day drifting in and out of consciousness wired up to painkillers and saline drips. My right breast felt tender but not nearly as painful as I'd expected. I was vaguely aware of nurses coming in and out through the day and night to check my blood pressure and wire me up to fresh bags of painkillers and saline.

Clooney arrived again at 7.45am the following day to show me my scars of which he seemed justly proud….a neat but jagged incision above my right nipple, a tiny incision under the right arm and some rather fantastic purple bruises covered by a huge surgical bandage. I could barely see the tiny dissolvable stitches, which meant there was no need to throw away my bikinis just yet. After a change of dressing I was discharged.

Iain arrived to collect me and handed me a bag with a sandwich and a bottle of water picked up en route. The relief on his face was palpable. The first part of our nightmare was over. Walking outside in the warm autumn sunshine with him, I felt amazing. We picked up my painkiller prescription, made an appointment for a week's time and drove home. After six weeks of living under a black cloud, it had just given way to blue sky.

The whole experience was made better by the fact that the French health service is an amazingly efficient organ. My hospital was clean, high tech, light and as cheerful as a hospital could be. It was rare to wait longer than 10 minutes for your appointment. On many occasions, I would arrive for a test or scan on time and a nurse or radiographer would be waiting patiently in the foyer to usher me in.

But a bit like pregnancy, when you spend months attending ante-natal classes to prepare for labour only to find it's a jungle out there once you've had the baby, the aftermath of an operation is the bit nobody goes into. I didn't know that the ridiculously strong painkillers I was sent home with were going to create the same kind of carnage as a week of eating vindaloo. The 1000mg tablets played havoc with my stomach to the point where I needed to be near a bathroom at all times. After several unpleasant blow outs I decided a little discomfort was infinitely preferable to a day spent sitting on the loo just in case and pushed the painkillers to the back of the medicine cupboard.

The house resembled a florist, with bouquets and cards everywhere, and the fridge was groaning under a mountain of organic dark chocolate (my request from visitors since finding out that dark chocolate, containing 70% cocoa solids or above, was better for me than milk or white chocolate. It contains antioxidants which help get rid of free radicals which can damage cells and in small amounts, it also helps to lower blood pressure).

Post op progress was slow but steady. On day one back home, I managed to put on my bra by myself and raise my right arm above my head. Doing everything with my left hand instead of my right was tricky. But somehow in the time it took Iain to take the girls to school and stop off at the boulangerie, I also managed to vacuum the house one handed (don't ask, there is a reason I was nicknamed Perfect.)

'What the hell do you think you're doing?' Iain shouted as he walked in from the school run armed with baguettes, croissants and coffee. I was standing on the stairs trying to balance the Dyson with my good arm while the right one hung uselessly at my side.

'Are you completely mental?' he raged. 'Go and lie down NOW.'

The cost of my nicely vacuumed ground floor was blood seeping through my bandage as a result of too much movement. The arnica had already brought out my bruising beautifully so I was now black, red and blue and so swollen that I couldn't even wear the sports bra, just a soft T shirt.

Having a shower and washing my hair was a big task all of a sudden, taking 90 minutes instead of the usual half an hour. I was only able to have a shower when the nurse came to change my bandage every other day, which isn't ideal for a girl who sweats on and off the tennis court, especially in 29 degrees of early autumn sunshine.

Peeling off the bandage, which was stuck to my nipple and the surrounding yellow and blue bruises, felt less painful when I allowed myself a few moans as I ripped off the adhesive. It hurt to lean forward as the pressure pushed against the stitches so I had to wash leaning slightly backwards, all the while trying not to slip over.

I looked at my reflection in the mirror. The scar was bigger than I thought...two inches circumference around the nipple, with an inroad incision into the breast at the top and bottom. But it was healing neatly and the rest of my breast looked normal, full, rounded and a bit perkier, just as Clooney had said it would.

Drying my hair for the first time post op by myself was another victory and not something I ever thought I would feel the need to write about. Exhausted after my first shower, I spent the afternoon in the shade on a sun lounger by the pool, sipping a cold glass of pink Veuve Cliquot with my girlfriends Milly, my savvy New Zealander fellow ex-pat who shares the same dark sense of humour as me and Sarah, my best friend from London who'd flown in earlier that day to check I was okay. I felt almost normal. After all the uncertainty and worry of the previous few weeks, it felt so good to be home.

And breathe….Don't overdo it. Think tough on the cancer but be kind to yourself.

Chapter Five

Chemo, The Big Bad Wolf

If ever there was a wolf in sheep's clothing, chemotherapy is it. Hard to believe that a couple of bags of innocuous looking fluid can take out the good, the bad and the ugly like some kind of hotshot super sniper randomly blasting everything in its path. The miracle is that it doesn't finish you off altogether, which is worth remembering when you're in the thick of it.

From the moment I was diagnosed with cancer, the over-riding thought in my head was whether I would be able to get well again without enduring the horrors of chemotherapy. Clooney had told me that he wouldn't be able to make a decision until he had the pathology report on the lump.

Chemo signified the worst case scenario in my head. It would be four and a half months of extra treatment when instead of getting on with my life, travelling, working, having fun and playing sport, I'd be sick, wired up to intravenous drips and would lose my hair, eyebrows and eyelashes.

The thing I dreaded most was losing my hair. I couldn't pretend that I wasn't bothered, however shallow that sounds. I tried to be brave but the thought of spending the best part of a year bald or tufty crucified me. It seemed so cruel that a disease which strikes at the heart of being a woman also had to mess with your locks.

When my lovely friend Lisa was dying of ovarian cancer and stressing about losing her hair, I told her: 'Forget your hair, this treatment will save your life.' Suddenly I knew exactly how she had felt.

Nevertheless, I was in buoyant spirits as I headed off to my rendezvous with Clooney a few days after surgery. The dull pain had subsided and I was slowly getting back to leading a normal life.

'Do you want me to come with you, babe?' asked Iain.

'No need,' I said breezily. 'It's only to check how I'm healing.' Somehow I was in denial about hearing anything other than yes, we've got it, you are getting better and by Christmas this whole deadly dull experience will be in the past.

I arrived at Clooney's light airy office decorated with paintings by French impressionists and we made small talk as he checked the scar and declared that it was healing well. Then he got out my notes, along with the pathology report revealing the test results from the lump and the three lymph nodes that were removed during my operation.

He looked up at me across his desk and suddenly I realised what a fool I had been to brush off the offer of some company. (Important: NEVER go to an oncology appointment on your own.)

'The lab found a small tumour in the third lymph node we removed,' he said cautiously. 'It's only 2mm but the tumour is Grade 2 not Grade 1, it's aggressive and faster growing than we thought. It has started to spread into your lymph nodes. I'm sorry we didn't pick this up during the operation.'

I felt my head spinning. So the scans and the tests during surgery had not told the whole truth. I should have woken up to the fact that the only way they really know what's happening is when they remove the offending bits and test them in a lab.

'Ok,' I heard myself say in a small voice I didn't even recognize. 'So what happens now? Does this mean I have to have chemotherapy?'

'Yes,' he said. 'I also have to do another operation to remove some more lymph nodes. Then you will have six treatments of chemotherapy, followed by six and a half weeks of daily radiotherapy.'

Somehow I managed to hold it together in his consulting room and ask all the questions I had flying around in my head that I hadn't even expected to need answers to.

'When can I swim in the sea?' I asked rather inexplicably as my first question. I'm not sure why this mattered – it certainly wasn't the most important question in my head – but suddenly it became very important to me.

'As long as you wear a waterproof bandage over your scar, anytime you like,' said Clooney, so my first stop afterwards was the hospital pharmacy to buy a packet of dressings.

'How big was the lump?'

'It measured 1.2 cms, so it was slightly smaller than the biopsy suggested, but it was growing at a rapid rate,' said Clooney. 'Some lumps can take five years to become a problem. Yours hadn't been there for very long.'

'What are the chances of recurrence once my treatment is finished?'

'Very low, and you can minimize that risk further by having your ovaries removed at a later stage. It's not something you need to think about just yet.'

I took a deep breath. 'Will I make a full recovery?' Clooney fixed me with a look.

'Yes, no question. The disease is localized, although it had started to move, but it will respond very well to chemotherapy and the radiotherapy will be the final fix.'

'Finally, I've planned a trip to Los Angeles next April, do you think I will be able to go?' I asked as my voice started to falter. We did some rough mental arithmetic between us to tot up chemo and radio treatments and his answer was yes. I shook Clooney's hand and left his office, whereupon the tears started to roll down my face.

I called Iain from the car and we cried our way through the conversation before somehow I managed to pull myself together and drive home. More tears were shed when I walked into the house and fell into his arms.

'I should have been there with you,' he said, fighting back the tears and hugging me as I wept. 'But at least they are throwing everything at you, which is a good thing.' We stood by the front door, hugging each other and trying to take it all in. I thought about how I would tell the girls and felt physically sick at the thought of giving them more bad news.

Issy arrived home and I told her my news. 'Mummy just needs one more small operation and then I have to have chemotherapy.' She looked bereft.

'Will you lose your hair?' she asked quietly.

'Yes, I probably will.' I adopted a jolly tone, adding: 'I haven't decided yet whether I'm a wig girl or a turban girl. Or perhaps I will just work the Star Trek look. What do you think?' She looked horrified.

'Mum, I can speak for both Liv and me when I say that we DO NOT want to see you in a turban,' she said sternly. 'Did you know there's a group on Facebook called ILSHMTFIMC, which means I Laughed So Hard My Turban Fell Into My Curry?'

She spent the afternoon morphing my head into new hairstyles on the net. Jessie J was too dark and severe, Cheryl Cole was too red, but the Cameron Diaz shaggy bleach blonde crop got the seal of approval. She's a cool, gorgeous surf chick so it was fine by me.

The race was on to find a wig shop before it fell out. Everyday frustration at the length of time it took to blow dry my hair quickly turned to relief that I still had hair to dry. I sent a plaintive text message to Milly, asking: 'Will you come wig shopping with me?' and she responded with: 'There is no-one I would rather go wigging with than you. And afterwards, we're going for lunch and a glass of Champagne, okay?' I wrote in my diary: 'Wig shopping PLUS CHAMPAGNE.'

And breathe…. Think positive thoughts as much as you can. Even when the world feels like it's turning against you, think of one good thing each day.

Chapter Six

Getting On With It

Leading as normal a life as possible was important for my sanity. Denial doesn't work for everyone but going to interviews and meetings and pretending to be fine was good for my morale. Equally, it was just as important to allow myself my down moments as the reality of having cancer hit home. Yes it's bloody unfair but the sooner you park the bitterness and injustice about being the one to get cancer, the better you feel.

Less than a week after the operation, I was invited to a press screening at the Mipcom TV Festival in Cannes followed by drinks afterwards with a very influential and powerful US TV contact at the Martinez Hotel on the Croisette. When I told Iain, he shook his head in disbelief.

'If your doctors knew you were doing this, they would go mad,' he said frowning. 'You are supposed to be resting at home, not rushing around Cannes working. For goodness sake, stop trying to overdo it. You don't have to be superwoman you know.'

'Look, I'll only be out for a few hours,' I argued. I omitted to tell him that I had also been asked to interview five actors from a new action adventure TV series called Missing.

I rifled through my wardrobe looking for something to wear that covered up the area where all my bandages were and didn't make me look like an extra from The Mummy. I settled on a cream crochet shift dress, which took 10 minutes to wriggle into as I couldn't raise my right arm to put it into the sleeve.

I felt nervous but somehow empowered getting into the car to drive to Cannes. It felt good not giving in to the bitch that was cancer although I was nervous about driving with limited movement on my right side. And once I arrived, it wasn't difficult to sit in a huge squidgy cinema chair for an hour watching an action-packed thriller.

Afterwards, I headed to the Martinez Hotel on the Croisette where my US studio contact, who lives in Los Angeles, was waiting in the bar.

'Hey Karen, how are you doing?' she beamed, as we did the bis (a kiss on each cheek) and I discreetly angled my right side away from her to avoid any pressure on my war wounds.

'Really well thanks,' I lied. I planned on sticking to fruit juice but couldn't resist a glass of Laurent-Perrier instead as a private toast to making it in one piece to my very first PC (post cancer) assignment.

We talked about work, mutual friends, her baby son and upcoming TV projects. What was really great, after weeks of talking about nothing else, was not talking about my health. It reassured me that my plan to keep my illness a secret from work colleagues was a good one, if only for the ability to answer the cursory 'How are you?' that starts every phone and email conversation with the white lie 'Fine thanks,' instead of 'Fine thanks, apart from the fact that I have cancer,' which is not what people want to hear.

The following day I drove to the Majestic Hotel in Cannes to interview Ashley Judd and her co-stars and producers in the hotel gardens. It was lovely to do something normal at a time when life felt anything but normal. Spending a few hours in the sunshine doing my job was a huge boost although I felt tired and in pain after standing around for short periods waiting to be ushered into each interview. No-one knew that I had just come out of hospital following life-saving surgery. I was just another journalist on the Croisette doing her job alongside thousands of others. In my eyes, I was Back on Top.

I stopped off at the hospital on the way home for a full body scan to check my bones and another breast scan. Both came back clear. Hurrah hurrah.

I interviewed Kathy Bates on the phone (instead of at her hotel in Los Angeles as had been planned BC) and she was a joy. She's a cancer survivor too, having been through ovarian cancer and breast cancer, which led to a double mastectomy, but I stopped short of telling her that we had something in common as it felt unprofessional.

Inevitably, after a few days of feeling invincible, also known as 'I have this cancer rubbish licked,' I had a low few days. The enormity of what was happening to me started to hit home and I became weepy and emotional, although I chose my moments and made sure the girls weren't around to see my tears. It was hard enough for Iain but he made it clear he was very happy to be a shoulder for me to cry on and confide in.

My instinct was to protect the girls the way my dad had protected me when he was diagnosed with a rare form of muscle cancer, Embryonal Rhabdomyosarcoma, in the mid-1990s. I was in my 20s, running around town enjoying a busy career in national newspapers when Dad was told he was terminally ill but I never saw him anything other than upbeat and positive right until the end, 14 months after diagnosis.

On the day Dad died, at the horribly premature age of 52, the whole family, including Liv, who was eight weeks old, spent two days in a vigil by his bedside in a London hospice. I was an adult with a young family of my own but I remember feeling helpless and hopeless and like a child again.

My dad waited until my brother Justin and I had left the hospice before he finally took his last breath with only my mum by his side. It was like he wanted to protect us from any more pain, and I now understood this, as my primary concern was making sure the girls saw me cheerful, upbeat and as damn near normal as possible. Protecting them and making everything seem okay went beyond any concern for myself.

After Dad died, his doctors told us that so aggressive was his cancer, he should not have survived four months beyond diagnosis. I know that wherever Dad is now, he is planning a different outcome for me. It's like having a guardian angel watching over you, sometimes his presence is so strong and I can hear his voice telling me what to do. He never complained once during his treatment, or asked why me, he bore it all with stoicism and courage. Without knowing it, he was a great mentor to me in how to get through the worst of times without letting them beat you.

My mum flew over from London to see me and although I felt utterly despondent, having her around meant I had to put on a brave face and carry on as I also wanted to protect her from the pain of watching her daughter fight the same disease that had claimed her husband. You end up trying to protect everyone around you, and as a strategy for carrying on and not giving up, it works. There is no concept of letting your loved ones see you beaten. If it weren't for my mum, Iain and the girls, this was a time when I could really have hit the buffers but having people look at me and see strength and courage helped us all to get through.

Dropping Mum at Nice airport was emotional as she didn't know when she would next see me or how I would look or feel. We both knew I would get an awful lot worse before I got better. Silly things made me feel desperately sad, like hearing Liv playing a lovely piece of music on the piano or Issy thrusting a piece of paper at me with the name and address of a wig shop that was recommended by her kind teacher at school.

I probably wasn't in the best frame of mind to start reading a self-help book sent by a friend entitled I Beat My Cancer: Let Me Show You How by Colin Ryder-Richardson. The title alone should guarantee you a seat on a crowded tube, in fact you could probably empty a carriage in no time at all. A lot of it was depressing but addictive in a what-the-hell-is-he-going-on-about kind of way. It talked of bringing on cancer yourself through your lifestyle, sex life or by being a negative or controlling person. I should point out it was written 30 years ago by someone who must be knocking on the door of 80, but who was still alive at least. Maybe the purpose was to make you so mad that you decide to disprove all the writer's theories by beating it your own way, in which case, it worked a treat. A better title would have been I'm a Bit Too Busy To Die Just Yet.

Many writers talk of how cancer changed their lives for the better.

I could never imagine saying that cancer was the best thing to happen to me. It was the shittiest thing to happen to me. When you eat well, exercise every day, don't smoke and generally respect your body, it's hard to think what kind of changes you could possibly make to your life. My lifestyle was certainly not a factor in me getting stricken by this very random, disrespectful space invader of a disease.

And yet I was learning lessons which would remain with me beyond my cancer battle. I could not remember a day in the year before diagnosis when I hadn't had at least one or two glasses of wine. I resolved to be more watchful about my alcohol intake in future.

I started reading Lance Armstrong's autobiography It's Not About The Bike. From the very start, it was so inspirational that I was shivering in the shade after my swim at the beach because I didn't want to put it down. Lance is a controversial figure since being stripped of his seven Tour de France titles following his admissions of doping while competing, but the fact remains that he has raised many millions of pounds through his cancer charity, The Livestrong Foundation, and adopted a determined approach to beating testicular cancer.

He talked about living fast and even sleeping fast, which sounded horribly familiar. Being forced to take my foot off the pedal and slow down a little was one good thing to come out of what had so far been a pretty crappy deal.

I didn't allow myself to think about losing my fight very often but I couldn't pretend that it hadn't crossed my mind in my darker moments. I knew Iain and the girls would be devastated if they lost me but I also knew they would get on with their lives and not allow it to destroy them because I had seen such strength from them all.

Apart from not wanting them to go through any more pain or loss, I wanted to stick around so I started planning my 50th birthday party. It will fall at the same time as I get the five year all clear so it will be a double whammy on celebrations, with a DJ, caterers, champagne, Moroccan tents in the olive grove and bacon sarnies at sunrise for the hardcore. Theme Studio 54, glamour all the way.

I came out of my black hole of despair by deciding that whatever else I did, I could not be a passenger on this journey. After days of moping about feeling sorry for myself, the Positive Mental Attitude came back following its tea break with the grim reaper.

And breathe…. Keep your sense of humour and laugh as often as possible. I didn't think it was possible to cry with laughter when you have cancer but it is.

Chapter Seven

You Are What You Eat

A little of what you fancy does you good. So do your bit, clean up your act and your fridge. Sugar is the enemy but you don't have to miss out. You can make your own cakes and brownies using healthy substitutes like spelt flour and agave syrup or xylitol in place of sugar so you can enjoy a treat without the guilt.

Before cancer, my diet was pretty healthy. I gave up red meat when I was 19 to follow a typically Mediterranean diet consisting of mainly organic fruit and vegetables, fish, olive oil, seafood and, since moving to France, herbs and fresh produce from my garden and that of Rosine, my elderly Italian neighbour, who grows pretty much everything.

Convenience food is frowned on in France and packet meals are fairly rare. Fast food equates to an omelette or scrambled eggs. Dairy and sugar were in short supply in our house. I only drank water (or wine). I wasn't perfect - I would grab a bag of crisps or a biscuit occasionally - but overall, I was pretty clean.

But hours of research seemed to point to the fact that a low acid, high alkaline diet would be my best chance of coming through chemotherapy, and cancer, in some kind of good shape. Evidence suggested that sugar, dairy, fats and animal proteins were more likely to encourage cancer cells to grow. Tumours are said to be sugar junkies and simply can't wait to shoot up on sugar in the bloodstream.

On my friend Angela's advice, I decided to consult Harley Street nutritionist Dr Simone Laubscher PhD, whose remarkable results advising diets based on your 'metabolic blueprint' to people with cancer could not be ignored. Granted, Angela in her heyday was the biggest party animal I knew but Simone had saved her brother-in-law from a bleak prognosis of leukaemia a few years ago so I was ready to hear more.

Her strategy is simple but effective. By eliminating the factors in our Western diet that overload the body, making it acidic and causing the digestive system to struggle, you free it up to work efficiently and effectively without too much strain. Making your body alkaline creates an environment that cancer hates and your system, which is already at full stretch fighting the disease and processing the drugs, is given a much needed break.

I had to fill in a detailed questionnaire about my eating habits, drinking habits (oh dear) and what I would really miss if I had to give it up, which was easy...chocolate, fish, seafood and Champagne. I also had to identify my goal, which was to get through chemotherapy feeling as well as possible, not to get sick during treatment and to make a full recovery.

My blood group O + along with my particular disease, age, lifestyle and treatment regime helped Simone to formulate a food plan which gave a nod to my favourite things while also arming me to withstand the toxic effects of chemotherapy and make my body hostile to further cancer growths.

It was radical but it made perfect sense: a mainly vegetarian diet rich in fruit, vegetables, berries, vitamins and minerals as well as the odd portion of seafood and fish which didn't deprive. I was allowed a free two course meal of my choice every week along with a couple of glasses of red wine or Champagne, which are less acidic than white wine or rosé.

My enemies were refined sugar, gluten (which can cause gut inflammation), dairy, alcohol (particularly cocktails, spirits, beer and white wine), meat and fats apart from olive oil and some nut and seed oils. Coffee was out as it is acidic and dehydrates the body. Instead, Simone advised starting each day with a pint of warm water with lemon and cayenne to detox the digestive system and kick start the metabolism – think of it as cleaning your teeth for your stomach. Interestingly, soy products, which are often used as a substitute for dairy, were also off limits for me, as they can mimic oestrogen which was what had caused my tumour to grow in the first place.

Bread was a big loss but I rose to the challenge of finding gluten free bread, known as petit épeautre or pain au seigle, at our local boulangeries, instead of crusty baguettes. I was never a big coffee drinker, one skinny latte a day was my usual habit, but giving this up was surprisingly hard especially as we had just bought a Nespresso machine which made the perfect cup of coffee. Replacing mangoes, which have lots of natural sugar, with apples was easier.

My friends were green tea, which replaced my morning cup of Earl Grey with milk (I'd read that three cups of green tea a day could significantly lower the risk of developing cancer and contains a fraction of the caffeine found in coffee or black tea), agave syrup (a natural sweetener three times the strength of sugar) and xylitol (a natural birch sugar which looks like regular white sugar and is an all-round wonder ingredient, with more than 300 studies indicating that it can play a significant role in preventing - and reversing - tooth decay). Basmati rice, gluten free pasta, nuts, line caught fish, plums, raspberries, sweet potatoes, spinach, broccoli and garlic also got the thumbs up. I was also allowed to eat goats and sheep products so halloumi, goats cheese and feta were all okay, as was sheep or goats yoghurt, which tastes like Greek yoghurt and is delicious.

Exactly a week after surgery it was my 45th birthday. I didn't feel much like celebrating. My mind wandered to the previous year when I was getting ready to go to Tokyo, and the year before, when I spent my birthday surfing in Malibu. But when you have two excited girls piling into your bedroom at dawn with a pile of presents and cards to open, you can't be churlish and hide under the covers, even if you want to. So we did the birthday thing, and I got some fabulous gifts of perfume, cash, jewellery, a beautiful leather jacket and an iPad from Iain so that I could read or work in bed if necessary. My best present was the one I gave myself, my consultation and food plan with Simone.

At my next hospital appointment, I asked Clooney what I could do to help myself. He said simply: 'Cut down on alcohol.' Perhaps the four most depressing words uttered since my diagnosis.

Everyone seemed utterly shocked when I announced I was giving up alcohol. Iain protested, saying, 'Well, the odd glass of wine won't hurt you, surely?'

My brother Justin was more shocked by this revelation than when I told him I had cancer.

'You're giving up alcohol? Forever?' he gasped.

Even Liv rolled her eyes and said: 'Hmmm let's see how long that lasts.' The last time I quit drinking was 13 years earlier when I was pregnant. Would it really be that difficult?

The first test was my best friend Sarah's weekend visit, a 48 hour swoop in from London to give me some moral support. Under normal circumstances, we'd uncork a lovely bottle of Champagne on her arrival and progress onto red or white wine at dinner. Instead, she had a few glasses of red and I stayed on water all evening. Surprisingly I didn't miss it. It was the ritual of uncorking a bottle and pouring a glass as I start making supper that I missed rather than the taste of alcohol. When I went to bed, I felt fine and a tiny bit smug in the knowledge that I would have a clear head the next morning.

No milk chocolate, cream or sugar, on the other hand, was proving a lot more difficult to stick to. As soon as you give something up, that is of course exactly what you fancy. Perhaps this is why so many diets fail.

I felt like a new member of Food Fads Anonymous. 'My name is Karen, I'm 45 and I'm a food Nazi.' Since my conversion to a non-dairy, very low fat, wheat free, sugar free, virtually caffeine free, teetotal (the only slight fail) diet, I had taken to patrolling the kitchen, checking the labels of everything I ate and obsessively making huge vats of soup to freeze down. I'd throw away any non-organic produce and hunt for evidence of banned substances like crisps, biscuits and cakes. I wouldn't let anyone touch my hidden stash of 70% minimum organic dark chocolate but if I caught Iain or the girls nibbling on Dairy Milk, I'd launch into an annoying lecture on the evils of refined sugar, white flour and saturated fats.

The family tried to respect my food fad frenzy but it wasn't easy. One evening, I started a huge row with Iain, who had sweetly offered to cook supper, over the amount of omega 3 oil he wanted to wilt the spinach in. Chez nous, I became known as 'The Nightmare.'

Nevertheless, he pledged his support, declaring to the girls: 'If your mum has to go through this, then the least I can do is keep her company on her food plan.' I might have believed him had he not uttered this while heartily tucking into a bacon sandwich washed down with pints of Guinness and champagne chasers during an England France rugby match.

I was also trying to economise wherever possible. Leftover vegetables were blended into soup or spiced up with turmeric and turned into curried pasties, too-soft bananas magically ended up as banana and walnut loaf and excess lemons from the trees in our garden made a perfect lemon drizzle cake. It wasn't as lucrative as writing features but it was a small contribution and made me feel slightly less useless about being unable to work.

It was frustrating that the very clean, modern chemo facility at my hospital, the Tzanck, had a vending machine selling soft drinks, coffee and chocolate bars when in my eyes, it should have been promoting water, green tea and fruit. I evaded temptation by taking in a flask of green tea and a home-made cereal bar on each chemo visit.

'How are you going to survive on this mum?' Liv asked on one of our first organic supermarket shopping trips as I piled our basket high with rice milk, cream substitute, omega 3 oil and a bar of dark chocolate. 'And can we have oven chips while you're in hospital?' Being so controlled around food was one of the most difficult challenges of Planet Cancer.

I started reading Anticancer: A New Way of Life by Dr David Servan-Schreiber, a physician and neuroscientist who, along with two colleagues, diagnosed his own brain tumour during an experiment in the 1990s. The book's thrust was about inhibiting the growth of bad cells and accelerating the growth of good cancer fighting cells through diet, positive energy and exercise and it resonated with me.

I was also inspired by Eat Right 4 Your Type, written by Dr Peter J D'Adamo, which outlines different blood groups and key foods to avoid, those to seek out and those which are neutral, so neither good nor bad for you. It also explains why certain body types have a propensity for developing cancer, heart disease and other chronic illnesses. In it, I found a passage about the CA 15-3 test, otherwise known as Carcinoma Antigen 15-3, which is given to monitor a person's response to breast cancer and indicate if breast cancer is likely to recur. The paragraph mentioned a woman with breast cancer whose tumour marker CA15-3 was 167. A normal reading is below 10. I raced downstairs to flick through my blood tests and found two sets of results....the first CA15-3 last September was 7.6, and the second was 8.1. Finally, a reason to be cheerful.

And breathe…. Cut down on alcohol. You don't have to give it up completely but the links between cancer and alcohol are well documented and shouldn't be ignored.

Chapter Eight

The Cold Facts On Chemo

There's a big support system around the big C. Psychotherapists, masseurs, reflexologists and beauticians are just a few of the people who can make you feel more human at a time when you really need a little extra TLCC (that's Tender Loving Cancer Care). Whether you walk the path alone or accept help from the people around you, just knowing the support is there can make a huge difference to your state of mind.

My next oncology appointment was with my chemotherapy doctor, Remy Largillier, who looked like a cross between a cyclist and a movie star. What is it with the French health service and their fit doctors? Maybe they moonlight for French Equity when they're not in theatre (the operating theatre that is.) This time Iain came with me and we discussed the next stage: a second operation to stop the carcinoma in my lymph node from spreading by removing five more lymph nodes in close proximity, followed by a heart scan and the onslaught of chemotherapy once every three weeks through the winter.

My cocktail of drugs was FEC-T, which is commonly used to treat hormone receptive breast cancer, and was split into two stages. We'd start with three treatments of Fluorouracil, Epirubicin and Cyclophosphamide. Spaced three weeks apart, they take two hours to administer but the party continues for the next few days at home with anti-sickness drugs, cream for sore hands and feet and mouth wash for ulcers. Fluorouracil is more commonly known as 5FU, which pretty much summed up my attitude to the whole scenario.

Afterwards, I would move onto the T in FEC-T, Taxotere, for the last three treatments. Dr Movie Star (who made the perfect partner for Clooney) told me I would lose my hair, although using the cold cap might mean being able to keep it for the first two months of treatment until Christmas. The cold cap is a system whereby the scalp is kept cool during chemotherapy, shrinking the blood vessels in the scalp so that less blood passes through them. The idea is that less of the chemotherapy drug reaches the hair follicles, which means the hair is less likely to fall out. It works for some people while others continue to lose their hair, just at a slower rate. All I wanted for Christmas was my hair but it looked like the E in FEC was going to put paid to that.

Movie Star seemed bemused by the idea that anyone should want to mask the effects of the drugs doing their job by expending huge amounts of energy trying to hang onto their hair. In France, it seems you just get on with it, you don't mope about it. It made me think of Laura Linney in the TV series The Big C, celebrating when her fingernails started falling out because it indicated that the drugs were working. I, on the other hand, would have been trying to Superglue them all back on again. Movie Star didn't know one patient who kept their hair through chemotherapy, so it seemed the egghead look was a done deal.

Other possible side effects included infections, neutropenia (an abnormally low count of white blood cells), anaemia, hypersensitivity, thrombocytopenia (reduced platelet count), neuropathy (nerve damage), dysgeusia (distortion of the sense of taste), constipation, anorexia, nail disorders, fluid retention, asthenia (loss of energy), pain, nausea, diarrohea, vomiting, mucositis (inflammation of the tissues lining the digestive system), alopecia, skin reactions, myalgia (muscle pain) and dyspnea (breathlessness). I felt breathless just reading the list.

We discussed the chances of cancer returning once treatment had ended and the conversation took a more cheerful turn. Movie Star swivelled his PC around to show me the medical website Adjuvant, a fabulous little tool which assesses all your criteria and delivers the probability of a patient developing cancer again after further treatment. Without chemotherapy, radiotherapy and hormone therapy, the chance of it returning rose to 36% over a 10 year period. But with those therapies taken into consideration, my chances of another cancer battle in the future dropped to 5%, which was a statistic I could handle.

I was weighed and discovered I had lost 3 kg through giving up dairy, gluten and alcohol. Forget the Dukan diet! We spent an hour with Movie Star, who seemed in no rush to get us out of his consulting room and patiently he explained the side effects of the drugs, chiefly fatigue, sickness, hair loss and mouth ulcers. Nice.

I left with a sheaf of prescriptions for potions and pills to pre-empt the worst effects and headed off to meet Sus, a lovely Danish nurse who would be looking after me during the coming months. Sus spoke perfect English and showed me around the chemotherapy unit.

If you didn't know it was a cancer centre, you could almost believe you were in a city hotel. Light, airy and clean, it was furnished simply and comfortably with large recliners, private cubicles with plasma TVs, a drinks machine, biscuit stash and a collection of leaflets offering holistic and complementary therapies, including Pilates classes specifically tailored to young women with breast cancer, a beautician to tattoo on eyebrows before they fall out, a psychotherapist to talk through any emotional issues and a support group in French and English, all provided free of charge apart from the heavily subsidized beautician.

The tour over, Sus asked: 'How are your children coping?'

'Well, it's hard for them...' I began and she interrupted: 'Are they in denial? Do they just want everything at home to be normal?'

'Yes, exactly that,' I sighed. The girls didn't ever bring up what was happening in front of me and whenever I tried to talk to them about it, they looked uncomfortable and couldn't wait to change the subject. All perfectly normal, according to Sus.

'Tell them they can come and look around the clinic with me if they'd like to see where you're being treated,' she offered. 'And if they have any concerns or worries they don't want to discuss with you at home, the counsellor is happy to see them and talk through their concerns.'

She suggested inserting the IV line to administer the drugs intravenously in the left side of my chest so that I could continue to play tennis with no fear of dislodging the line.

I left the clinic feeling for the first time like I was walking on air. Sus assured me that after the first few days post-chemo, I'd have two weeks of feeling pretty normal when I could work, travel within reason and lead as normal a life as possible. Even our long-planned pre-Christmas trip to London was given the green light despite falling slap bang in the middle of my third chemo treatment.

'We can push it back by a few days,' offered Sus when I tentatively told her of our travel plans. 'We can't bring it any closer than 20 days between treatments because your blood count won't be high enough. Sometimes we have to push back a few days anyway for this very reason, which is why you need blood tests a day before each chemotherapy, to check the white blood cell count is high enough.'

This was music to my ears as the original date would have meant having my fourth treatment the day before New Year's Eve. Having it a few days afterwards meant that even if I was slumped in a chair in a corner bald and wrapped in pashminas, I would be able to celebrate New Year's Eve with a hopeful heart and get stuffed full of drugs again in early January, when the rest of the world would be sleeping off hangovers, overdrafts and rubbish weather. Amazing, the things that please you on Planet Cancer.

And breathe…. Say 'no' more often. No-one will argue with you and you will never have a gold plated excuse like this again to get out of anything you don't fancy doing so USE IT!

.

Chapter Nine

Team Chemo

My natural state is optimism but I found that learning to expect the worst meant that I was no longer having my hopes dashed so a smattering of pessimism became the order of the day. And sure enough, in the case of chemotherapy, while there is no denying that it was bad, my first treatment was actually nowhere near as bad as I had anticipated.

Slash, poison and burn: that is what they call my treatment regime. First it's surgery, then chemotherapy, then radiotherapy. If I'd known how well me and hard drugs would get on during chemo, maybe I wouldn't have been such a coward in my youth!

My second operation to remove five lymph nodes had gone to plan and two weeks later, the day I had been dreading - my first chemotherapy treatment - arrived. It occurred to me as Iain drove me to hospital that instead of them, the poor sick people with cancer, and me, it was us. I'd become one of them, although I wasn't ready to admit it. I was shown to a comfortable booth with a recliner and a chair for a companion, although I had decided to go it alone and gave Iain permission to make himself scarce.

I noticed a tall, handsome man in his 40s heading to the next booth with his elderly dad in tow. How sweet of him to come along and keep his dad company, I thought. We said hello and I took in his elegantly casual attire and distinguished air. Then I saw his dad wander out for a coffee half an hour later, unencumbered by a drug trolley, and realized that he was there to watch over his son during chemotherapy.

The doctor checked me in, consulted my heart scan, blood tests and radio scan of the IV line and I was wired up to the drip for the first FEC infusion. It was strangely uneventful and less momentous than I had imagined. They stuck the needle into the catheter buried in my chest, which I didn't even feel thanks to the local anaesthetic patch I'd been wearing, and I was away.

Sus explained that I would probably feel okay for a few days while taking Solupred, a corticosteroid which modifies the body's immune response and decreases inflammation, but once I finished each dose three days after chemotherapy, I would feel tired.

I reminded her about the cold cap and she returned with a soft blue plastic padded helmet, the infamous ice cap. It looked just like a crash helmet filled with ice, or one of those comedy caps you wear when playing the bungee jump game.

'I can't promise this will save your hair but we can try,' she said. She sprayed my scalp with cold water to make the cap more effective and then placed it on my head. It felt cold but not totally unbearable, a bit like holding a cold shower on your head or doing a headstand in the Arctic Circle. For two hours.

I'd heard terrifying stories of how awful the cold cap was, how some people gave it up after 10 minutes. I remember thinking: 'Well, it's not pleasant but surely it's going to get worse than this?' But it didn't. Compared to the pain of my first labour, a 23 hour forceps delivery followed by 40 odd stitches, the first round of drug therapy paled into insignificance.

Afterwards, I felt a bit of a fraud. I was woozy and lightheaded but it was nothing like as bad as I had expected. If I could get through feeling a bit squiffy for the following four months, I would be very happy.

Each morning the following week, I woke up expecting the worst but apart from the slightly metallic taste and a small wave of nausea, I felt almost normal. The five anti-sickness tablets I was taking daily were clearly working. I rested, ate soup and slept pretty well apart from the odd two hour insomnia episode in the middle of the night, a common side effect of the treatment.

I walked the dogs in warm sunshine, shopped at the health food shop where I became a regular customer and spent afternoons baking with Issy using my healthy new sugar and flour substitutes, agave syrup and spelt flour, which meant I could eat the delicious ginger cake and pumpkin and nut loaf that we made guilt-free.

Two days after chemo, I went for my first run in a month. I started off a bit sluggish but picked up my pace, pausing only to fast forward The Verve's The Drugs Won't Work, and made it back four minutes over my usual time of 30 minutes. Having run marathons, half marathons and 10k races, in normal circumstances a 5k run wouldn't be a stretch but it felt every bit as good as completing my first London Marathon and was the best high I'd had for quite a while.

I was convinced the reason I felt so good was thanks to the diet. I will never know for sure how much of a role it played versus my natural physical strength but giving up coffee, cream and the other substances Simone had banned was a small price to pay for feeling good. My local nurse Anne rang to check how I was doing and sounded surprised when I told her. 'Genial!' she exclaimed.

I started to make a massive effort whenever I left the house to pre-empt the prospect of people seeing me looking anything less than glam and thinking, 'Poor Karen, since she got ill, she really has let herself go.'

Previously, my daily beauty routine was a splash of water on my face (yes, I know, dreadful) followed by moisturiser and a quick brush of powder to take away any shine. The new regime took three times longer; cleansing, moisturising and performing home facials twice a week, in addition to rubbing bio oil into my scars to help them fade and also into my fingernails and toenails, gargling religiously with mouthwash to prevent mouth ulcers and rubbing glycerin cream into my hands and feet to stop my skin drying out.

I tried to keep moving, playing tennis, going running, even oiling the garden furniture by the pool. I emailed a friend who said: 'What on earth is in your diet? I need to give my husband some. I asked him to take down the parasol at the end of September and it's still out there being buffeted by the wind and rain!'

I did not want to come across as anything other than completely in control. I met up with friends who were very complimentary about my hair and how well I looked. I was going to make damn sure I didn't look anything less than on form. It was tiring keeping up appearances but it was a legacy of the BC Perfect Karen era and had to be done.

One of my Fleet Street gang was particularly perturbed at the many plans I had made for their eagerly anticipated visit a week after my second chemotherapy. My four oldest journalist mates, who I had met in my early 20s when we worked together at The Sun, had planned to come and stay in the hope of cheering me up and onwards through the next few months. I suspected that they also wanted to check that I was still breathing.

I called Sally a few days before their arrival to outline all the things I had lined up. I was mid flow when she interrupted in a high pitched wail.

'Hang on, I thought we were just going to lounge around at your house, in our PJs, eating chocolate, chatting, drinking tea and watching boxed sets? You shouldn't go rushing around you know.'

'No, I'm fine, I feel great at the moment, so we might as well get out and do lunch and explore a bit,' I persevered, a bit too keenly for Sally's liking.

'But Karen, I'm really tired, I just want to chill out with you,' she said. 'I'm really happy not to do anything at all. I'm only packing PJs and track suit bottoms.'

I had to laugh. My friends viewed coming to visit me as an opportunity to get off the treadmill for a little while and just be. No plans, no deadlines, just log fires, boxed sets, nice snacks and long lie-ins. I, on the other hand, saw their visit as a beacon of light, a social whirl in an arid desert of early nights, no drinking and generally living a blameless, boring existence.

Whenever I felt myself getting a bit down, I would think about Marika, a beautiful blonde Swedish pilates instructor who was introduced to me by my yoga teacher Faye. Five years ago, she was diagnosed with stage II breast cancer aged just 36. You would never believe that such a vivacious woman (with a huge mane of blonde hair) had been through this horrible disease. She had also lost every hair from her head and body.

I knew we were going to get along brilliantly when she said: 'You know, when people talk about cancer being the best thing that ever happened to them, I have to wonder what on earth they are talking about. It's one of the worst things that can happen to you even if you do learn lessons from it. The thing you have to remember after it's all over is to not slip back into the habits you promised yourself you would break.'

'Hmmmm,' I pondered. 'I mean, if getting cancer is the best thing that has ever happened to you, your life must have been pretty rubbish up to that point!' We both fell about laughing. She also talked of how she felt totally betrayed by her body, which summed up my feelings too.

The best news I'd had in a while was hearing that two girlfriends in the UK got the all clear after their biopsies. They had only booked mammograms as a result of my bullying and neither was expecting to need further tests. I cried with relief when I heard their good news and I cried a few tears for myself and the fact that their results weren't mine too.

And breathe…Increase your intake of water and other alkaline fluids like herbal teas, as chemotherapy causes the body to dehydrate. You will also feel as if you are flushing the drugs through your system if you drink more.

Chapter Ten

My Hardcore Eating Plan

Propping up your immune system at a time when drugs and disease are wreaking havoc on your body has to be a good thing, right? On a practical level, forget eating five a day, you need to double that, hit the vitamins and minerals and embrace probiotics and milk thistle. You might be surprised to find how much you can still achieve. On an emotional level, if you want to confide how you're feeling to all and sundry, do it, and if not, that's fine too. Remove all pressure. There's no right or wrong way, just your way.

When you are first told you have cancer, your world ceases orbiting. Holiday plans, work assignments, social engagements and family commitments stop in their tracks and suddenly your life from that moment on is dictated by doctor's appointments, tests, scans and treatment. Losing control feels alien when you are used to running your life with devastatingly accurate precision. So being able to make a difference to the way your body behaves and handles the disease and the treatment, by paying close attention to how you nourish and care for it, is a way of regaining an element of control.

Just under two weeks after I started Simone's food plan, we Skyped and I did a urine test to see how my body was dealing with all the trauma, drugs and changes.

'You are low on minerals so we need to load those up and although one of your liver markers is happy, the other isn't, so we need to support your liver more,' Simone explained. 'You also have a parasite living in you, which isn't unusual with cancer, so we are going to get rid of that.'

It's amazing what one pee stick can tell you about the workings of all your vital organs but I was a bit deflated by the news.

'There is good news too,' she added. 'Some people have five to 10 areas that we need to work on straight away but you have just four, which means your body is working well overall,' she added. 'And your kidneys are doing a good job.'

Extra 'cocktail' ingredients were prescribed: 100% organic supergreens with spirulina, chlorella, barley and wheat grass, milk thistle tablets to support my liver, Ark amino acids, a probiotic capsule to kill the parasite and Cellagon Aurum, a German super tonic containing dozens of vitamins, minerals and other goodies. I mixed it up and it was unlike any cocktail I have ever drunk before, sludgy green in colour and tasting only marginally better than it looked, which was like pond water.

It was too tempting not to order a latte macchiato at a café in Vence on a shopping trip with Liv, although she had to restrain me from quizzing them about what kind of milk they used. I ate the mini chocolate they brought with it and tucked into the apricot and almond tart I couldn't resist buying at the patisserie. As I had been such a spectacular rebel, Liv insisted on paying with her new cash card. I tried to argue but she wouldn't budge. She wanted to celebrate my fall off the gluten free bandwagon.

The rebellion continued that evening when I tucked into chicken and prawn curries, bombay potatoes, flatbreads, nougat and chocolate, washed down with Laurent Perrier rosé. All on the same day Simone told me I was her star pupil!

By late November, my blood counts were faltering, which was par for the course two chemos in. Falling asleep in front of the television at 9pm became the norm so I started on a course of GCSF injections, three spaced out over a week immediately after chemotherapy. Granulocyte Colony Stimulating Factor, to call it by its full name, is a growth factor that stimulates the bone marrow to make more white blood cells. The first injection gave me a headache but the second passed without any problems. It was reaching the point where a week without appointments, chemo treatments or injections felt as good as winning the lottery.

The third jab was administered by a nurse I hadn't seen since she came to change my dressing just after the first operation. She didn't recognize me at first and then asked: 'Have you lost weight?' When I told her I had shed four kilos, she shook her head, adding that I needed to make sure I didn't lose any more.

One morning as I got out of bed to get washed and dressed, I noticed a hardness of tissue just under my skin on my right breast, the site of the first operation. The skin above the scar was also puckering a little. I tried to get through to the Macmillan helpline – a great source of practical information for all things cancer - but got stuck at the very polite voicemail telling me they were extremely busy. In desperation, I rang Clooney to ask whether I should be concerned.

'It's perfectly normal,' he assured me after I described my symptoms. 'As long as it isn't swollen, or red or painful, it isn't an oedema. It will disappear in the next month or two. Apart from that, how are you feeling?'

'I can't believe how well I am,' I told him. 'I've had no sickness, very little fatigue and I'm running and playing tennis again. I'm just concerned that my next chemo won't be as good as this one.'

'You mustn't worry,' he said. 'The first treatment is like a test, to see how your body copes. It should mean that you continue to feel the same all the way through the chemotherapy. There's no reason why you should get a different reaction next time.'

You have to love the science of doctors. They only deal in hard proven medical facts, not anomalies or one offs, so to say I felt like uncorking the Moet, despite it being 9.30am, was a rather large understatement. I told him all about the blood group diet and he listened patiently while I rambled on about how I thought it was making a difference.

'It's an interesting idea,' he admitted, which was about as close as anyone in the medical profession had come to telling me that it might actually be a good thing. I was turning into Delia Smith, baking sugar free cookies and apple and pear crumbles. I was eating close to 12 portions of fruit and vegetables a day which accounted for why, 10 days down the line from the first chemo, I still felt fantastic.

Torrential rain meant I couldn't go running for a while as the chemo was wiping out my immune system so I had to wait until warm sunshine returned before venturing out for a half hour gentle jog. I let my iPod play on shuffle and listened to great tunes that sparked memories of carefree fun. Calvin Harris's Ready for the Weekend and Eric Prydz's Pjanoo reminded me of Sarah and I getting ready for a mad night clubbing in Cannes (the anticipation was actually better than the reality, which was hundreds of 17-year-olds getting wasted on vodka and Red Bull to a soundtrack of thumping electro dance music). And the Ting Ting's That's Not My Name recalled a pizza party night when the adults danced round the house to the amusement of all the teens.

I desperately wanted my old life back but as that was impossible, the example set by Jennifer Saunders, who was diagnosed with breast cancer in 2009, was the one I wanted to follow. Her illness wasn't a well-known fact, her friends knew but the public didn't and she just got on with it quietly and privately. When she felt rough, she didn't go out and when she felt okay, she ventured out in her wig. Her story was an inspiration and felt like a similar situation to mine, with many of my work friends and colleagues completely in the dark about what I was going through. It meant I could have a chat about interviews or the weather without my health being the dominant topic of conversation.

And breathe… Cut down on as much refined sugar, gluten, fat, dairy and meat as you can (especially during chemotherapy). I was not sick once during treatment and I feel strongly that reducing the above played a key role in keeping me well during drug therapy.

Chapter Eleven

It Will Grow Back

Losing my hair was the hardest part of my cancer battle. Some people put a brave face on it. It's only hair, they say, it will grow back. But other friends who have had cancer felt the same way as me. I hated my alien, moonfaced appearance and being literally stripped bare. It's painful for me to write this even now. Cut your hair short, my doctors told me, then it won't be so traumatic when your hair starts to fall out. That's a big fat lie. Losing your hair is hugely traumatic; it saps your energy and your self-esteem. You look older, more fragile, more sick. But the people who love you can still see your beauty and strength shining from within.

As an every-other-day washer of hair, it didn't come naturally in chilly November to postpone washes to every three or four days in freezing cold water in the hope of persuading my follicles to stick with me on my journey. I had been warned that around two to three weeks following my first chemo, my hair would start to fall out.

On the night I was diagnosed with cancer, I threw away the last dregs of shampoo and conditioner in the shower and grimly ripped open the expensive new colour care products I'd just bought with the cheerful thought that I might as well use them straight away in case I died! Two months on from diagnosis, it had become a question of whether I would get to the end of the bottle before my hair started hitting the plughole.

Every morning, I checked the pillow and the plug, searching for tell-tale hairs. I'd give my hair a big hearty tug just to make sure it was still attached. It was like hearing the scary music in a movie and knowing that some horrible fate was about to befall the heroine at any moment. The scary music was playing loudly and I was waiting for the bogeyman to leap out from behind me waving a handful of blonde crop.

A fortnight and one day after my first chemotherapy, I was idly running my fingers through my hair when tiny clumps started coming away from my scalp limply, without a fight, a dozen hairs at a time. The exodus had started. I felt more depressed than at any point since diagnosis. Bucking the odds and not becoming a baldie was no longer an option or a hope. My lady garden was following suit and starting to shed and the hairs on my legs, which would usually be stubbly after two days re-growth, seemed to be growing back much more slowly.

My hairdresser Charbel must have heard the desperation in my voice when I called him to ask if he could wield some scissors on what was left of my hair. In the space of eight weeks, I'd already seen him four times. In September, four days before my diagnosis, he had cut, coloured and curled my hair for the Monte-Carlo party with the beau monde.

The second time, I went from long to a short unstructured bob (after Sus and Movie Star had urged me to go short to minimise the trauma of losing it. They meant well but trust me, it minimized nothing.) In fact, what was more frustrating was that I really liked my new style which made everything seem even more grossly unjust as it was not going to last beyond a week or two. Sure enough, Charbel had to return a few days later to redo my highlights as what was left was very dark and unflattering, before finally coming back to chop the straggly remainders - around 50% - into a very short crop.

The only positive was that while in my long hair days, not washing it frequently would've meant it looking horrific by day three, cut short it seemed to behave better the dirtier it got.

I showed Iain the loose clump of hairs in my hand and he hugged me, telling me: 'Well, at least we know the drugs are working.' I told the girls and asked if they were interested in seeing me bald. Liv said yes, Issy said absolutely not.

'I'm going to text you every day when I get off the bus from school,' she added, 'and you need to make sure that by the time I walk into the house, you are wearing your wig. Okay?'

Milly and I laughed about Issy's five minute warning as we set off on our wigging expedition to a shop that was recommended by my hairdresser. We flicked through brochures full of wigs, hairpieces, turbans and scarves while we waited for the proprietor to finish helping an elderly customer. Most of the styles were straight out of the 1950s – all that was missing was an apron and a gin & tonic with an olive on a stick - and we tried to muffle our laughter as we picked out the most horrific ones on offer.

I wasn't totally filled with confidence when the dear old lady in her 80s left looking like she had a family of ferrets perched on her head.

'Jesus, please don't let me leave looking like that,' I pleaded with Milly as we fought back the giggles.

I spent an hour trying on different wig styles and with each wig I tried on, more and more of my own hair fell out. It felt like it was giving up the ghost and admitting defeat which was the part that angered me the most. If I wasn't giving up and holding cancer's hand, why was my hair? The assistant examined my head very gently before breaking the news that I had maybe another week, two at the most, before my hair was completely gone, which made the wig decision process even more critical.

There was only one style that came close to looking halfway normal, the Thais. It was the wrong shade but shared the same name as one of the key characters in The Killing so it seemed like a good omen. I left empty-handed, telling the shop assistant I would return a few days later when she had the Thais in the right shade.

To cheer myself up, we headed for lunch to my favourite Italian restaurant in Cannes, where I ordered spaghetti vongole made with gluten free pasta. We commiserated about the lack of wig choice for anyone under 80 with a few glasses of Prosecco and a cheeky coffee before heading to the rue d'Antibes, Cannes' answer to Bond Street, for a morale boosting clothes buying frenzy.

As predicted, virtually overnight, I was moulting like a hairy labrador trapped in a greenhouse. My clothes were permanently covered in loose strands and piles of hair lay all over the house. A few days and a few thousand hairs later, Liv and I went back to the wig shop so I could try on the Thais in the right colour. Issy set off for school that day unimpressed at the fact that her big sister was getting a day off school to come shopping with me, until Liv set the record straight.

'I'd rather go to school every day for the rest of my life than have to shop for wigs with Mummy,' she told her sadly, which brought tears to my eyes. Both of them had been amazingly stoic and brave and had matured so much but I would have given anything for them to be their usual carefree selves again.

Liv gave the Thais the nod so I bought it even though it wasn't really me. Let's face it, no wig was going to be me so I also bought some lovely suede sheepskin boots which were very much me to cheer myself up. When I got home and tried it on in front of everyone, Liv was effusive while Iain was quietly cheerful. They were both trying hard to say the right things. Issy shook her head with a sad look on her face and said she supposed she'd get used to it before going upstairs to her room.

I followed her upstairs and asked her if she was all right. She nodded but her eyes glistened with tears.

'I don't want you to lose your hair and I don't want you to have to wear a wig,' she sobbed.

We had a cuddle and cried together and I assured her my hair would grow back eventually.

'Don't ever be afraid of being honest with me about how you feel,' I told her. She found some photographs from our summer holiday in Puglia that she had been looking at and pointed at me with long blonde hair, saying: 'This is how I like you to look.' She later confided that seeing me with short hair was the first time it really hit her that I was ill.

I promised I would grow it longer as soon as I could. It was just another thing to hate about Planet Cancer. Why should a little girl have to be brave? It wasn't fair and my heart was breaking for her. She should have been having fun, not worrying about me. I grabbed the dogs and headed out for a walk and a good cry.

The wig sat on its stand in my bedroom, patiently waiting for the moment I could no longer get away without it. I tried to avoid mirrors because staring back I didn't see me but a fragile, straggly haired old woman with lines.

On the plus side, I hadn't felt really unwell and I knew I could deal with the hair loss although I had no idea that it would be this aspect of cancer, rather than two operations and a stomach full of toxic drugs, that would depress me the most.

When I arrived for my second chemo, the first thing Sus said to me was,' How come you still have some hair?'

'I've lost a lot but maybe the cold cap is having some small effect,' I told her.

'Well, I thought you'd have pretty much nothing by now, so let's keep going with it,' she said cheerfully. Weirdly, this boosted me more than I can explain. Anything to avoid the dreaded wig, which following a trim from Charbel now resembled a cross between Suzi Quattro and the Bay City Rollers. He's a great stylist but wigs are not his forté.

A pattern was establishing with chemotherapy. I felt woozy a few hours after, a little nauseous on the second day and then pretty good for the remaining two and a half weeks before the next treatment. We even managed to go to dinner with friends in Monte-Carlo 24 hours after my second chemo, which gave me a chance to forget about my hair traumas for a while and enjoy beautiful food and funny conversation.

It was funny conversation which was helping to keep me going. My preferred method of chatting to friends was on Skype, although why I was up for a video chat with anyone when I couldn't even look at myself in the mirror was a mystery to me.

And breathe…Buy the best wig you can afford. There are some horrors out there and looking like an extra from One Flew Over the Cuckoo's Nest will not help when your body image is already at an all-time low.

Chapter Twelve

Keeping One's Chin Up

In normal circumstances, there's nothing I love more than a house full of visitors. Feeling down and under par, it was tempting to retreat from the world and see no-one but being forced to talk to visiting friends and neighbours who would pop by for a morale boosting green tea and a chat was good therapy even if I didn't always feel in the mood. Sometimes you don't know when your spirits need lifting until someone comes along and does just that.

My four oldest Fleet Street journalist buddies rolled into town just at a time when I really needed a lift. I had several cold sores around my mouth and a permanent metallic taste inside it. Everything had become a huge effort, even getting out of bed to shuffle to the bathroom was slow, painful and left me feeling breathless. If anyone could pull me out of the black hole that was swallowing me, it was the little gang of four I had spent my early 20s working with: Clare, Sally, Angela and Sarah M. As we sat around chatting with cups of tea (green for me, PG Tips for the girls), Angela produced a bag from her case with the nicest blonde wig I had ever seen, donated by a friend of hers, a fellow breast cancer survivor in Suffolk who I'd never met.

We held our own Leveson style inquiry fuelled by Champagne rather than tap water and Iain said it was just like having his mates to stay, except mine were louder, drunker, more coarse and vulgar than any of his friends.

Despite the way I felt and looked, the girls kindly suggested that I was faking it to get them to visit. They returned to London completely exhausted after bracing walks, coastal lunches, shopping expeditions and late night suppers. The only blip was chronic food poisoning following a fishy lunch at the coast, which left me thanking my lucky stars that the effects of my chemo were not the same every three weeks.

There was good news and not so good news at my next appointment with Movie Star. My white blood cell count - which usually hovered somewhere between 4,000 and 10,000 - was on the lower limit, which was more usual at the end of chemo than the beginning and meant a high risk of infection. But oh joy, the five lymph nodes removed in the second operation were given the all clear.

The physical effects of chemo were well underway, my immune system was low and the cold sores weren't budging. My morning routine turned into boot camp, including careful combing of the virtually non-existent hair with a wide tooth grip as a brush removed too much hair, swilling with mouthwash to prevent mouth ulcers, applying cream on the cold sores and bio oil on my scars, using CFC and aluminium free deodorant, then careful application of make-up to disguise my very tired looking face. I had gotten used to the stares from old people and small children as my scalp was on full display every time the wind blew and bloody chilly it was up there too.

I was defiantly refusing to wear a wig until absolutely necessary. The cashmere beanie that Sally bought me when she visited with Fleet Street's finest wasn't worn for fear of taking away precious hairs each time. On the way to tennis, Liv and I bumped into our neighbour Rosine, who has a habit of saying exactly what she thinks. She told me that I looked thin and tired in her heavily accented French.

'Charming,' said Liv, 'and then you went and told her how well she looked!' Well, she did look better than me, there was no denying it. Just when everything felt like it was getting too much, I was offered a fabulous job in Toronto, interviewing Elle Macpherson and the finalists on the Sky Living show Britain and Ireland's Next Top Model. By happy chance, it happened to be planned around the end of my radiotherapy so I had a fresh incentive to badger my doctors to speed my treatment along. It came at just the right time as I was starting to feel very despondent. Christmas was rapidly approaching, and with it invitations to meet up with friends for drinks, soirées and nights out but getting ready to go out and realising that even a comb over was no longer effective and the Touche Eclat was nowhere near enough of a touch to cover the cold sores was a grim realisation.

It didn't matter how many people told me I looked great (considering), all I could see on the days I was brave enough to look in the mirror was someone 20 years older, fragile and exposed. And that was at the start of the Christmas party season, not the end.

My mum suggested not going out at all but that seemed like a sure fire way to feel even more depressed, particularly as France does such a lovely job of Christmas, with white fairy lights festooned on every palm tree, roundabout and high street, festive markets in every town, carol concerts and snow on the nearby mountaintops.

I took to wearing high heels whenever I left the house, so that only people over 5ft 10 inches tall could see my bald patches and toyed with the idea of hanging around with dwarves.

The dreaded third chemo loomed and after the blood tests showed the all-important white cell count to be 5,000, as opposed to the very low 4,000 on the second chemo, I met Movie Star, who noticed straight away that I was thinner, at just under 48 kilos, or 7 stone 5 lbs. He gave me a well-meaning lecture on how to keep my weight up but frankly he was preaching to the converted as I hadn't weighed so little since my teens and it was not a good look on a 40-something.

The problem lay in the fact that after chemo, the very last thing I felt like doing was eating. I had about two hours before going downhill to the point where my appetite was at a standstill for two or three days, during which time not even lunch at Gordon Ramsay's could have tempted me.

Movie Star moved onto the menopause, telling me that around 75% of women having chemotherapy start the menopause early. If the chemotherapy doesn't put you into it, the Tamoxifen does. In an interview with the Radio Times in December 2011, Jennifer Saunders talked about feeling depressed at the mood swings and hormone imbalances that Tamoxifen caused during her treatment for breast cancer. 'You are pushed into menopause like jumping off a cliff... bang!' she said.

Funnily enough, the idea of the menopause didn't bother me. One of the few highlights of major drug therapy was the prospect of my periods ending. In November, I was three days late which was unheard of, and in December, six weeks after chemo started, I was a week late. By the following month, there was nothing, which felt like a small reason to celebrate. No more cramps, being caught off guard or using smelly loos at the beach.

Annoyingly, given the sparsity of hair on my head, my leg hairs were still impertinently poking their heads through, albeit a lot slower than usual, and the tiny soft blonde hairs on my arms were also hanging in there, unlike the lady garden which was looking very pruned and sparse. How is this fair, I wanted to ask.

I headed off for the halfway point chemo armed with my iPad to answer a few work emails, make some pitches for work commissions and line up some interviews. It felt surreal tapping away about filming schedules while intravenously wired up to bags of toxic fluid. As I left, I spotted two surgeons fresh out of the oncology operating theatre still in their scrubs rushing through the double doors to the communal gardens to light up cigarettes, which was even more surreal.

I had a grotty two days of feeling completely rubbish, heady and tired although thankfully I was not sick. I told Iain I wished we didn't have so many mirrors around the house, because catching sight of my reflection made me shudder at the thin, old-looking shadow I had become.

'Don't say that,' he pleaded. 'You're still beautiful. It's what's on the inside that counts. And the way you look now only means that you are getting better.'

By day three I started to feel a bit better. Swallowing up to 16 tablets a day, some of which were so big that they made me heave, didn't help the nauseous feelings but I managed to wrap some Christmas presents and sit at my PC for an hour. I mused on the pluses of cancer and came up with two: No blood shot eyes (due to barely drinking and no late nights) and being back at the weight I was at 17 (although it was not such a good look on a bald 45-year-old).

On day four after chemo, I felt well enough to do the school run. On the way home, I met Rosine and her elderly friend and as we chatted, I relayed to them how much hair I'd lost. As we headed down the drive, Issy said: 'Only two corrections today mum but the first is quite important...you were talking about losing your horses NOT your hair...it's cheveux not chevaux, okay?'

And breathe...Order all the boxed sets you missed out on first time around for the days and nights when facing the world is beyond the call of duty. The Killing and Curb Your Enthusiasm kept me sane.

Chapter Thirteen

Working It

In times of crisis, work has always kept me going. I love my job and the perfect day for me is juggling lots of commissions and interviews, planning exotic assignments abroad and ultimately, delivering good copy.

Before we had children, Iain often came home from a long day in the City financial markets to find me ensconced in my office at home in North London, toiling away on an interview using only the light of my computer screen, oblivious to the fact that the house was shrouded in complete darkness. I have always had the ability to lose myself completely in work no matter what else is going on.

So to go from a crazy schedule that took me all over the world to cancelling jobs left, right and centre to allow for my trips in and out of hospital felt surreal as well as bloody unfair. I decided from the start to keep my illness a secret from all my work colleagues apart from Clare, Sally, Sarah M and Angela.

To the rest, I cited a clash of commitments. My colleagues must have thought that I was the busiest writer in the freelance world because every time a great job came up, I would tell them that much as I'd love to say yes, sadly I was too busy to commit. It was frustrating and I felt bad about lying to them, but it would have been much harder to tell the truth, explain everything and leave them thinking that Karen was either going to spend the next year in bed, or worse still, not be around for much longer.

I didn't want pity, or people thinking I was too ill to be bothered with phone calls or emails about upcoming jobs. Like my girls, I was in a little bit of denial about having cancer and felt that if I could keep it a secret from colleagues and work contacts, then I could carry on like nothing was wrong. And when it came to the crunch, I still had bills to pay and wanted work to be the one area of continuity in my life. Being freelance, I didn't want to risk commissioning editors writing me off and no longer offering me work.

I soon realised it was naïve to think I could carry on working at anything like a normal pace. A diary chock-a-block full of doctor's appointments and tests is not conducive to racing around at the drop of a hat and getting on planes to go and do interviews. Just before Christmas, I was offered a job in Cuba, interviewing Benicio del Toro, one of my all-time favourite actors, only to find that it clashed with chemo. I wrestled with my desire to go to Havana versus the amount of juggling I would have to do to persuade the doctors to change my appointment. The added risk of being so far away from home if anything went wrong was another factor, so very reluctantly, I decided it was safer to turn it down. It was one of the few times when I felt very sorry for myself and cried at the unfairness of it all.

My other concern was what people would think when they saw me. I always made a huge effort whenever I was going out on an interview to dress up and look my best. That was now impossible. I was skinny and pale with thinning sparse hair and there was nothing I could do to disguise that. It seemed unfair to rock up at a meeting or interview acting like nothing was wrong and expect people to act normally and not stare or ask questions.

I decided my safest option was to say yes to phone interviews only, which I could do from home without moving from the sofa and no-one would have to see me. I developed a technique for subtly checking out whether an interview was a face to face or a phoner and once I had established it was over the phone, I would check my busy diary and magically discover that I was available after all. These phoners were few and far between, however, because I didn't feel I could hustle for work like I usually would in case it turned out that it clashed with yet another hospital visit.

I tried to keep as busy as possible when I wasn't attending appointments, reading all the papers on my iPad, researching yet more anti-cancer wonder ingredients and clinical trials, reading cancer forums and keeping a diary about what was happening to me and how my body was responding to treatment.

Not working and watching my earnings dwindle to nothing was not good for morale. I'd earned my own money since starting a Saturday job in a pharmacy in Highgate, North London, at the age of 14 and had worked full-time through both my pregnancies. I was used to a frenetic daily pace so to go from a career that was at full throttle to virtual standstill was difficult. Finance was an added pressure for Iain, who felt he had to keep all the balls in the air, concentrate on his lighting design business, cover all of our household expenses singlehandedly and make sure that I had nothing to worry about other than getting well. Physically and mentally, he found it an enormous challenge and scaled down his business trips to the UK so that he could cook, clean and play mum and dad to all three of us.

On the days when I was too tired to run or walk the dogs, I would doze on the sofa, surrounded by my iPad, books, magazines and mobile. It was no life for a busy girl about town. I stopped using Twitter and Facebook virtually overnight as I had nothing of interest to post. I tried to keep my blog chirpy but general and vague with no mention of illness, and updated it far less than usual.

The only upside to not working much was that in the girls' eyes at least, I was actually a better mum. Issy told me: 'You know mum, you are much more sociable and chatty now because you're not always on email, on the phone or writing on your PC. The only thing I don't like is when I look on your iPad and see loads of cancer tabs open, or find lots of cancer books lying around the house.'

My cover was blown a month after my treatment ended when a friend innocently posted a photograph of me on Facebook at a music festival completely bald. I received a flurry of concerned emails from work colleagues as far afield as Australia asking if I was okay. But by this time, I felt I could be honest about my illness with everyone because it was in the past and I was getting stronger and looking better by the week. I still think it was the best way forward for me, just getting on with it quietly and privately and with as little fuss as possible.

Looking back, I'm sure I worried unnecessarily as my wide network of fellow journalists are just about the most decent bunch of people you could wish to meet. But word travels fast in my business and the idea of being 'poor Karen who has cancer' did not appeal.

And breathe....My iPad became my most treasured possession and my constant companion. It allowed me to source endless research, make to do lists, read the papers, stay informed and even watch TV in bed when I was too tired to sit downstairs. Every cancer patient should have one.

Chapter Fourteen

Christmas Spirit, Anyone

A breakout of cold sores is never a good look, especially during Christmas party season. I started taking L Lysine and vitamin C supplements on the advice of my nutritionist and stayed away from eggs, chocolate and peanuts, which are high in the cold sore causing ingredient arginine, and there was a marked improvement. Planning a New Year's Eve party at home (when for once I didn't feel guilty asking friends to bring food and Champagne) was also a morale booster.

They say Christmas is right up there with divorce, death and moving house in terms of stress. I'd never understood this before, being the big kid who embraced all things Christmassy. White pea lights festooned the terrace, I'd choose the biggest pine tree we could fit in the house and we'd wrap up for the charity carol concert in the village, singing and sipping mulled wine in the frosty night air.

This year was different. The girls were up in arms about the fact that I hadn't bought a real tree and I heard myself making excuses...we were going to London, then I'd be having chemo, then I would be low on energy...but the truth was, I just didn't want to go and choose one and decorate it with Christmas carols blaring and mince pies in the oven, as was our usual ritual. My heart wasn't in it, I was finding the forced jollity a struggle and I was rubbish at pretending otherwise.

The only good thing was the house was a stress-free zone, instead of the usual mad fest of scribbling cards, shopping and wrapping gazillions of presents. There seemed no point in sending cards containing my miserable news to people I hadn't seen or heard from in a year so I didn't send any.

We received a Christmas newsletter from some old friends in the UK wishing us happy holidays and telling us about their year. It made me realise that mine would read quite a lot differently from their tale of GCSE successes, school trips and family holidays.

'Hello, happy Christmas and here is the Kershaw's news from 2011. Iain is busy working like a dog juggling Skype calls, taking orders and barely finding time for a wee while I take it easy, meet friends for lunch, recline on the sofa watching chick flicks, take drugs, spend money I haven't got and walk the dogs.

'Issy has perfected a beautiful scowl over the last year and only uses it when things don't go her way, which is most of the time. Her favourite sport is goading her sister, she excels at this and indeed if they were prizes to be won, she would be an Olympic world champion. Liv spends virtually all of her spare time in bed, daydreaming, pretending to do her homework and occasionally venturing to the bathroom for a wash or to the fridge for a light snack. She is getting much better at moving about the tennis court but has yet to win a Wimbledon title.

'The dogs enjoy chasing the cats and making their lives a misery, barking at every visitor and generally lazing about living the life of Riley. Ditto the cats, who also enjoy walking on newly changed bed sheets with muddy paws and disembowling the odd rat for me to trip over outside the back door.

'Travel has figured large this year. Karen swanned around in Miami, New York, Florence, Rome and London living the high life, lunching with friends, lying on the beach and generally doing pretty much what passes for her job until cancer stopped her in her tracks and Iain has made a few trips to Dartford and Norfolk on urgent international business.

'So all in all, a jolly busy year, what with trying to beat a life threatening illness, avoid bankruptcy, hang onto my hair, finish doing up the house and keep the peace. Here's to you and yours and 2012.'

Iain had bought the girls an iPad each and everyone else was getting a Selfridges gift card. My one concession was watching The Santa Clause movie with the girls. They forced me and I have to confess that secretly I enjoyed it.

After an attack of guilt at the Bah Humbug I had become, I hunted out the star garland, the red berry wreath, the LED Christmas tree, the eco fairy light tree and old St Nick in a bid to make the house look festive but not even Nat King Cole and Wham's Last Christmas could shift my mood. If I could have hidden away under the bed covers until January 1st 2012, I would have gladly done so.

I fell off the nutrition wagon in major style with the temptation of Christmas snacks and goodies. Six weeks' worth of champagne (or 12 glasses, somehow that sounds less shocking) were demolished far too easily in the space of three days, along with copious biscuits and Heston Blumenthal mince pies.

To cap it all, pardon the pun, I had the most horrible hair humiliation in Nice. I decided to pick up some Prosecco at Galeries Lafayette but had to park the car by the beach as the car park was full. The winds were so strong that a weather warning had been issued and the windsurfers were scooting across the bay at breakneck speeds.

By the time I'd walked from the car to the shopping mall, my hair was standing on end like I'd been plugged in at the mains, with bald patches clearly visible all over my scalp. I had to leg it to the refrigerated wine cabinet to stare in the tinted glass door at my chaotic appearance and try and pull off a comb over with my fingers whilst other Christmas shoppers looked on in surprise.

By that evening, I decided that fighting the moulting onslaught was a completely useless waste of energy. I shuffled upstairs, feeling defeated, and took the blonde wig off its stand, plopped it on my head and went back downstairs.

'Hey, it looks great but you don't have to wear it around the house,' said Iain, so I took it off and left it on the arm of the sofa, at which point Issy walked into the room and said: 'Mummy, why aren't you wearing your wig?'

For the first time ever, I could see my scalp. It was like looking at a moonscape, paler than my face, with a few freckles and a couple of moles I didn't know I had. On the plus side, it was smooth and a nice shape if I had to be bald.

Being reminded of how I used to look was becoming painful. I was browsing through photographs on my camera when I stumbled across some taken a couple of months earlier of me with long, healthy, glossy blonde hair. I felt the tears pricking at my eyes. Liv said: 'Mummy, your hair looks great short but can you grow it long again once this is over? You used to look like a prettier version of a wag.' I think she meant it as a compliment.

I went running for the first time in my newly designated sports wig (aka the Suzi Quattro number) and my beanie. With a hat on, I looked fairly normal and for once I didn't get any pitying looks. However, the builders renovating our pool were convinced that Iain lived with a harem...I left the house in my plugged in rocker's wig, came back and channeled the bald look for a while and then went out shopping in my slightly more chic ash blonde number. My hairdresser Charbel sent Christmas presents to all of us...hairbrushes for the girls and, sensitively, a coffee flask for me.

At least my cold sores were improving thanks to Simone's advice and the great news following my pee test was that all my markers were moving in the right direction. My mineral and vitamin count had gone from very low to optimum, both liver markers had improved and the parasite count had improved by 50%. I was still too acidic - perfectly normal for someone having chemotherapy - and dehydrated, so the water intake had to increase. But I'd moved from 4/10 to 6/10 despite a few cheats which I guiltily confessed to.

'It's Christmas, you're bound to slip up here and there,' Simone told me. 'If people are cooking for you, make sure they stay away from gluten and sugar, everything else is manageable.'

Simone was thrilled with my pee. 'Your urine results have put a big smile on my face,' she told me. 'Everything is going up which is great news and you have had the fastest response to the diet and supplements I've seen in my cancer patients.

'In fact, you're doing so well that I'm going to give you a Christmas present of two days off over Christmas and two days off over New Year to kick off your shoes, drink Champagne and have fun!'

I can't pretend that I wasn't thrilled at the prospect of living a little more on the wild side despite the fact that whenever I slipped up, I felt sluggish and bloated and my digestive system felt under strain. When I was good, it behaved and did its job efficiently and productively. Feeling such marked differences made me want to get it right more often than wrong but being given the green light to go a bit crazy was the best present I could have wished for, especially as we were about to depart for our pre-Christmas trip to London.

In the lounge at Nice airport, I ordered a glass of Champagne and lived dangerously in the snack section, grabbing a bag of ready salted crisps. Airport lounges used to be the worst part of travelling for me, especially if I had to loiter for hours waiting for connecting flights, but I realised how much I had missed them after not flying for five months. The 100mph gales on arrival in the UK played havoc with Miss Wiggy, so I had to hang onto my hair as we disembarked on the rain lashed runway but it was a small price to pay for being back on home soil with my friends and family, who made a huge fuss of us all.

We returned to France and had a quiet Christmas at home. I managed to get through it fairly cheerfully but keeping a smile plastered on for 48 hours to reassure everyone via Skype that I was okay was no easy task. My hairdresser friend Karin arrived from the UK on Boxing Day with her scissors and somehow managed to make my two wigs into presentable versions of me, as well as trimming the remaining bum fluff stray hairs left on my head.

My mood faltered when I heard the sad news that Sue Carroll, an old Fleet Street colleague I worked with at The Sun, had lost her battle against pancreatic cancer. Sue was the most glamorous, funny writer and executive at The Sun, a brilliant tabloid journalist who could be caustic and no nonsense but who deep down had a very kind soul. She always had time for a chat and her throaty laugh used to reverberate around the office. I emailed her some months earlier after reading a moving account she had written about her cancer battle in The Mirror. Her death felt horribly close to home.

To take my mind off things, we went skiing to Isola and, for the first time in ages, I felt alive. Skimming down the slopes under blue skies in bright sunshine, life felt a little bit good again. I managed three hours of skiing but noticed that the frame of my sunglasses really pinched my head where there was no hair to cushion my scalp.

On New Year's Eve, surrounded by friends, who arrived laden down with home-made curries and copious quantities of Champagne, we kicked 2011, three chemos and four months of treatment in the butt and raised our glasses to a toast of 'Good riddance.'

And breathe….Swap wine, beer and spirits (all of which are quite acidic) for Champagne (which is less so). You'll be drinking less alcohol anyway so it's not a false economy. And invest in one of those bubbly corks so you aren't tempted to finish the bottle!

Chapter Fifteen

Battling On

Sometimes it's good to know when you are beaten. I was willing to try most things, including wearing an ice cap to try and save the last of my hair. But putting on sub-zero ice gloves and boots to freeze my finger and toe nail beds in the hope of preventing my nails from falling off was an agonizing step too far. The treatment is harsh enough without putting yourself through additional agony so I didn't feel bad about quitting.

Following the second operation, the mobility in my right arm was severely affected, with bizarre raised rope-like tendons standing proud under my arm and all the way along the inside of my elbow and down to my wrist. Stretching my right arm out fully, the pain and disfiguring ridges ran from scar to wrist. When I pointed it out to Movie Star at my fourth pre-chemo rendezvous, he advised me to book an appointment with a physiotherapist.

After 20 minutes of painfully manipulating my arm on a massage bed at her practice, the physiotherapist Nathalie established that my muscles had gone into protective mode following the operation and were clenched and immobile, creating the rope effect down my arm, a condition known as Axillary Web Syndrome, or Cording. It affects around 25% of women after a lymph node operation, sometimes it clears up and sometimes it lasts for years. After the first session, I stood up and for the first time in three months, I could stretch my right arm fully without feeling shooting pains.

'We have some work to do but it is normal for the muscles to react like this after an operation,' said Nathalie. 'They are in trauma so we have to release them slowly and gently.' She warned me not to do too much, adding: 'I don't know you well but I can tell you are a busy person who likes being on the go. That was your old life, now you have to slow down and think about your health and do the things you enjoy but slower. Don't be hard on yourself.'

Fiona, who had been a tower of strength since my diagnosis, offered to drive me to chemo and we went to the lab to pick up my blood test results en route. They were disappointingly low. My white blood cells were just 3,500 and my red cells, which should have been between 4.5 and 5.7, were 4.09.

Dr Hoch at the chemo unit prescribed an injection called Neulasta for the final three chemotherapies, to help build up the blood cells more quickly than the GCSF jabs by stimulating the bone marrow. I asked the chemist if I could take all three injections home at the same time but he shook his head. 'They cost €1132 each, and have to be refrigerated so I can only give you one at a time.' Together with a pack of Emend anti-sickness pills and the three Granocyte injections, my pharmacy bill that day came to €1600.

Fortunately, my status as an auto-entrepreneur, or self-employed sole trader, and the fact that my business was registered in France meant that I was in the equivalent of the French NHS and my all-important Carte Vitale, or healthcare card, meant that all my drug and operation costs were covered. If this hadn't been the case, my treatment costs would have run into many thousands of euros.

I spoke to Dr Hoch about my looming trip to Los Angeles for the Coachella festival, surfing and the job in Toronto with Elle Macpherson.

'It's really important that I take this job because I haven't worked very much at all for three months,' I pleaded. 'Can I start having radiotherapy and chemotherapy simultaneously and get it over with a bit quicker? Or start radiotherapy just after chemo ends?'

'No we can't do that because the combination of drugs and radiation is too toxic,' he explained. 'Your white blood cell count needs to be higher. But I want you to be able to work so let me ring your radiotherapy doctor and find out if we can bring forward the radiotherapy so you don't have a three or four week break before it starts.'

I listened in on the conversation and heard him saying: 'She is young and she is doing really well with the treatment.' But the answer was a resounding no, because the toxicity of the chemo too close to radiotherapy could cause problems.

'We 'ave to do a certain dose of rayons,' Dr Hoch explained patiently in very broken English,' if we condense it into too short a time frame, it will be bad for your breast, it will look, how you say, ugly.' That should have been enough to shut me up. It wasn't.

'Okay, can you tell him I am very fit, I'm going running two days after chemo, not lying in bed throwing up for a week at a time,' I continued. 'I'm prepared to take a hit on feeling rubbish for a couple of weeks if it means I can go away in April. Pleeeaaase!'

'Leave it with me, I will talk to him again and come back to you.'

He arrived half an hour later with a big smile. 'It's okay for LA,' he beamed. 'We will win back a week by pushing your last two treatments closer together. It's exceptional but we can do it.'

Thank you, I love you forever! What about Toronto?' I persevered.

'Maybe not, but you can go to LA.' One out of two wasn't bad but Sus listened intently and said she would fight my corner to make them both happen, adding: 'I can't promise anything but I will try for you.'

The worst moment in what had already been a very stressful morning was still to come. To head off the side effects of the new drug Taxotere and protect my finger and toe nail beds, I needed to start wearing ice gloves and boots for each chemo session. They came straight out of the deep freeze with the ice steam still rising. The cold cap was bearable but as soon as I put the socks and gloves on, the pain was intense straight away. Imagine digging through snow with bare hands and feet and you have some small idea of what it feels like. Within a few minutes, my fingers and nails were throbbing with an intense pain that is impossible to describe. Fiona watched the colour drain from my face and tried to keep me talking but I was writhing in agony. My fingers were a blue-ish purple colour and swollen to the extent that my wedding and engagement rings were cutting into the flesh.

After 15 minutes, I was close to collapse. I couldn't concentrate or hold a conversation but I was loathe to give in and remove them altogether. A worried Fi called Sus over, who said: 'Just take them off for a few minutes and put them back on again.' Once I took them off and the feeling slowly started returning, it was even more painful.

'Don't do it darling, you've tried so hard already, it's not fair,' said Fi, looking distressed as she put the ice gloves to one side and placed her soft warm leather gloves on my hands before placing them under her armpits to warm them through. Sus arrived and shook her head.

This is no good, we won't do the gloves again.' She sat holding my hands and rubbing them gently. It was the first time since the last operation that I had been in such physical pain. I could feel tears pricking my eyes. If the nails were going to fall off, fuck them, they would grow back, and it would be a good excuse to go to London and see the brilliant nail technician who rebuilt my toenails after I lost them running the London Marathon.

I had enjoyed rapid bounce backs post chemo so it was a shock to discover that I was as human as the next person. Following the trauma of the cursed ice gloves, it was a relief not to feel nauseous and heady after Taxotere but the Neulasta miracle jab, which replaced my thrice weekly Granocyte injections as a super blood cell booster the day after each chemo, was a real bugger. The leaflet in the box warned that aches and pains were a likely side effect but nothing prepared me for what was to come.

Less than 24 hours after the injection, it was an effort to lift myself off the sofa. My lower back, my head, my hips and legs felt like throbbing lead weights. The pain intensified to the point where the gentle run I had planned in the warm sunshine seemed as likely as climbing K2. Getting out of bed was a major operation, never mind walking down the stairs. I felt like I had been run over by a lorry and it made me realise that I'd had it pretty good so far in terms of avoiding the physical debilitation caused by my treatment.

The girls downloaded movies to my iPad so that I would sit still and somehow I managed to bake a gluten free, sugar free banana and walnut loaf by propping myself up against the kitchen work surfaces between mixing (the word mental comes to mind.)

Being prone and immoveable had no advantages whatsoever as far as I could see apart from the obvious fact of letting your body heal. My physio warned me not to do much on my right side and as a result of paying attention and quitting the I-can-still-be-Superwoman vibe, the mobility in my arm improved further and the hard scar tissue around the first incision on my right breast became soft and supple again. It pays to listen to the experts.

And breathe....Being part of the decision making process with treatment made a huge difference to my state of mind. Squeezing the treatments together, once I knew it was safe to do so, made me feel that I was jogging a little faster down the seemingly endless tunnel I was stuck in.

Chapter Sixteen

Even The Eyebrows?

I was looking less like a woman and more like E.T....wrinkly, bald and just to complete the look, my eyebrows and lashes started to fall out too, having hung in there until a few weeks before the end of chemo. 'Where's the justice in losing them now?' I wanted to scream. But all you can do at this stage is wish the last few weeks of treatment away and make plans for when you are looking and feeling better. And accept (and apologise for) the fact that you will be bloody difficult to live with for a while.

I'd reached a point where managing a whole day without painkillers was difficult. My usual 20 minute walk with the dogs along our quiet country lane had turned into a major challenge but the only thing worse than getting off the sofa was not getting off it.

My taste buds were completely shot. My mouth felt like a cat dirt tray that needed emptying. The roof of my mouth was dry, rough and scaly and I had a permanent bitter taste of iron filings that overrode even the strongest of flavours. I tried to reawaken my sense of taste with two pieces of Christmas cake and a piece of banana and walnut loaf (well, that was my excuse) but it was like chewing cardboard.

My teeth felt like they'd been pulled from my gums and there was a constant dull ache inside my mouth. My lips were cracked and peeling like old wallpaper, my teeth looked discoloured and the stubborn cold sores put in a reappearance. And thanks to the bone marrow injections, my legs felt like they had been pulled out of my joints and placed beneath a lorry full of gold bullion. In the night, I was suffering from a hacking cough that made me sound like a 60 a day smoker.

Despite feeling tired and aching all over, I dosed myself with painkillers to take the dogs for a walk with Iain and have lunch on the coast. We stopped at a restaurant in the marina and I noticed two kids drinking red grenadine, which looked just like one of my IV chemo drugs. I kept willing myself to stay positive and fight the feelings of negativity that were threatening to engulf me but my fragile mental state was making me quite tricky to live with.

Iain was invited out for supper to celebrate a friend's birthday and the news that he was going out put me in a foul mood which even I was at a loss to understand. He had been working flat out and hadn't left the house for weeks. I hated myself for having a problem but couldn't keep the note of fury out of my voice when he told me. He was in a lose-lose position because although I had no energy to go out, could not drink and all food tasted bitter and unappetizing, rendering the idea of a few glasses of wine and a curry about as appealing as swimming the Channel, I didn't want him to go out and have fun without me.

'Look, I'm only going for a few hours, I won't be late,' he said as he was leaving. 'We can always go out together on Friday night for a bite to eat if you fancy it.'

'I don't want to go out,' I said miserably. 'What's the point? I look terrible, I can't taste anything and I don't even fancy a glass of wine.' I omitted to add: 'But I don't want anyone else to go out enjoying themselves either.'

Watching everyone getting on with their lives without interruption was the crux of the problem. Losing the freedom and desire to do nice things was taking a toll on me. And because I couldn't do nice things and enjoy life, no-one else was allowed to either without me feeling hard done by. It wasn't fair and I felt selfish. I had to work on my misplaced sense of injustice.

The new me boasted gaunt features, a greyish scalp (who knew you need to wear foundation on your head so that it matches the colour of your face), a waxy skin that proclaimed 'serious illness' loud and clear and bones jutting out all over the place. That is what I saw when I looked at the naked me in the mirror. The curves I once had were gone, replaced by sharp angular lines. Where my thighs used to meet, you could see broad daylight through the gaps. My wedding, engagement and eternity rings were jangling loosely on my fingers and my watch almost slid over my hand completely without undoing the catch. I had to make new holes in my belts and my skinny jeans no longer hugged my butt but hung limply.

The disease, along with the prolific treatment regime, had stripped me back to bare bones. It isn't always the case. Two friends who ate their way through chemo believing that they would lose weight in the way cancer often dictates found they were 10 kilos overweight at the end of treatment and had to sign up to boot camp to shift it. This was one problem I wouldn't be having.

I hated looking so weak and thin. Most of all, I hated looking like a middle aged bank teller in a bad wig. I was particularly tuned into the way people behaved around me. At the supermarket as I packed my shopping at the checkout, the cashier called to her colleague sitting opposite. I glanced up sharply from my bags, expecting her to gesture at me, perhaps because she had noticed I was wearing a wig. I had noticed her staring at me on previous shopping trips. She caught my eye and said, 'Don't worry', to her colleague, which just confirmed my suspicions that she was about to talk about me in French.

The demon on my shoulder wanted to shout: 'Yep, take a good long look, IT'S A WIG! Would you like to see what's underneath?' And then whip off my hairy friend to reveal my shockingly bare scalp. But that would have caused a bit of a commotion if she was just asking for a new till roll or some extra carrier bags. I found myself hoping that anger was a good emotion because I had endless supplies of it.

I was getting ready to go out with friends for supper when I noticed my eyebrows had started dropping out, along with my eyelashes. I only needed to brush my hand past them and little hairs came away on my fingertips. I grabbed a brown Mac eye pencil and shaded them. It was pretty amazing how much fuller they appeared with just a little help. The dilemma with eyelashes was whether to avoid wearing mascara as taking it off meant losing more precious lashes but not wearing it made my eyes look sunken so on it went on the odd occasion I had somewhere to go and the energy to make the effort.

It was nowhere near the emotional trauma of losing my hair, however, because I was too tired to get worked up about it. Nothing would ever be as chilling as that feeling of hairs lightly landing on bare shoulders.

I had to stop running. Only for a short while, I told myself. I felt tired all the time. It was a given that I was asleep on the sofa by 9pm every evening. Despite the lack of energy, I did my first job in three months, a phone interview with an LA based Disney actress and it felt so good to use my brain for something other than counting out tablets or planning hospital appointments.

I needed things to keep me going so I started researching Cap Ferret on the French west coast for a surfing break. The very idea of carrying a board along the beach or struggling into a wetsuit was beyond comprehension but I had to believe that life as I knew it BC was going to resume in the future, however much of an impossible fantasy it seemed on those long cold days in January 2012. Every week that dragged by was taking me closer to the finish line, as the dozens of encouraging emails from friends and family assured me, but most of the time, it felt like a very steep, dark, lonely climb in the wilderness.

All my life I've been competitive. I refuse to give up or go for the soft option and it's not always my most attractive quality. I remember Liv, aged eight, running a mini marathon in Hertfordshire with the rest of her classmates at school. I was the mum 200 metres away from the finish line shouting myself hoarse at her to go faster, even though the winner had already crossed the line. She staggered towards the ticker tape before collapsing into a heap of tears and exhaustion. She has never forgotten it, or let me forget it either. To my girls, competitive is a dirty word, and their constant refrain was: 'Mum, stop being so competitive. It's the taking part that matters. Why do you always want to win?' But that extraordinary desire to win was the very thing that was now keeping me going.

Before cancer, I was a perfectionist. My articles were finished well before deadline, my house was immaculate, my children ate a proper breakfast every morning before school. I'd go off round the world on lovely assignments and arrange for our cleaner to come the day before I got home so that however chaotic things got while I was away, calm, order and clean sheets ruled from the moment I put my key in the front door. If one of these things wasn't as described, I felt like a failure. None of this is normal, or particularly common, or even comfortable to live with. Maybe it's why I earned the nickname Perfect. The time had come to let go of perfection. Simone had told me that being a perfectionist was not a bad thing as long as you also indulged your inner rebel.

I went to see my friend and dogsitter Helen, who had just had breast reconstruction following a mastectomy two years earlier. I arrived with almond croissants and pain aux raisins from the local boulangerie and we tucked into full-fat lattes as we talked drugs, how to beat the blues, how soon you can safely start to work out again after surgery and all the other niceties of cancer treatment.

She told me about an American woman at boot camp who came up to her and said in a reverent hushed tone: 'Are you one of the survivors?' Helen was confused but once she worked out that the woman meant cancer survivor rather than the reality show kind, she nodded, at which point the woman started rubbing her arm vigorously like she was a talisman or a rabbit's foot, saying: 'Well done for making it this far. I'm hoping some of your luck and strength will rub off on me!'

There were times when I felt like a poster girl for cancer. If someone had a friend who had just been diagnosed, I was the go to person, which was fine if you were in the mood to talk about it but sometimes I just wanted to forget it was happening and gossip about clothes, parties and inane rubbish.

I've had conversations and asked and answered unpalatable questions that I would never dream of sharing with someone outside the Cancer Club, not even my family, in fact especially not my family. All your loved ones want is for you to get better; they cannot countenance worst case scenarios, death or suffering, and don't want to talk fear, just hope. It was better to protect them from the darker conversations.

Helen and I talked about our fears of not being around to see our kids grow up. Not an easy conversation to have with anyone but it was a relief to be brutally honest with someone in the same situation as me. Neither of us were under any illusions that cancer could come back in the other breast, or reappear elsewhere, and the only thing we had going for us was that we were more aware of subtle changes in our bodies and the doctors would be scanning us at regular intervals.

I found myself making deals with a God I was not sure I believed in. 'Please God, give me 10 more years to see the kids properly grown up. Actually, please God, can you make it 20 so I can see them get married and meet my grandchildren? I wouldn't mind 30 years but I'm aware that would be a massive bonus so I won't hold you to that.'

I thought about what I wanted at my funeral....no black, lots of colour, no tears, Natural Woman by Aretha Franklin and Life on Mars by David Bowie, a lovely reading by someone erudite who could make the congregation laugh about what a great girl I was followed by a bloody fabulous party afterwards somewhere amazing with the best Champagne. Some arum lilies would be nice too but no other flowers, just donations to a breast cancer charity. Then my ashes could go to Cornwall to my dad's favourite beach, St George's Cove, near Padstow, to be scattered by my family across the same beautiful bay where we scattered his ashes 18 years earlier. And only then would they be allowed to cry.

And breathe…Set yourself small, achievable goals each day (even if it's just brushing your teeth on the bad days.)

Chapter Seventeen

Keeping Informed

Talking to my doctors, asking questions and keeping up with the changes in my body had become a full time job. It wasn't made any easier by my failing memory, another common side effect of chemo, but thankfully this was a temporary problem that would subside after treatment finished. Well, that was the hope.

One of the biggest dilemmas when you are diagnosed with cancer is whether or not chemotherapy will help your long term survival. At lunch with friends, I met Isabella, who had recently had a mastectomy and had been given the Oncotype DX test to decide if she needed chemotherapy. This radical test was news to me but is commonplace in America and Isabella's surgeon at the Memorial Sloan-Kettering cancer hospital in New York advised her it was a good idea.

The Oncotype DX test is a breast cancer test that looks at the activity of 21 genes within a woman's tumour sample in order to provide an individual probability of the likelihood of breast cancer returning in women with early-stage breast cancer whose tumour is oestrogen-receptor-positive and lymph-node-negative, or in post-menopausal women whose tumour is lymph-node-positive and hormone-receptor-positive. In addition, the Oncotype DX test provides information about how much benefit a woman is likely to get from chemotherapy in addition to hormone therapy.

Some patients are borderline cases, in which case a doctor may advise opting for chemotherapy just to be safe, not really knowing whether it will improve chances of survival or prevent a recurrence further down the line. I started off as one of these cases. My Ki-67 reading - based on the protein in cancer cells that increases as they prepare to divide into new cells - was 20%. In breast cancer, under 10% is considered low, 10-20% is borderline and above 20% is considered high.

My surgeon initially advised me that I was a borderline case for chemotherapy depending on the pathology results but he knew that my lump was fairly recent and that the cells were dividing at a rapid rate. Once they found the tiny carcinoma in one of my lymph nodes, the die was cast on me needing chemotherapy, raising my chances of long term survival by a significant percentage according to Adjuvant, the medical website used by doctors and patients in the UK and around the world to assess the risks and advantages of further therapy after surgery.

But in Isabella's case, with no lymph node carcinoma and a cancer that was Ductal Carcinoma in Situ (DCIS), the medical jury was out on whether chemotherapy would help her. Movie Star recommended chemotherapy to her as a preventative measure but after running the Oncotype DX test, which costs around $8,000 in America, it was decided that she wouldn't benefit greatly from chemotherapy after all.

I found it incredible that someone who had had a mastectomy didn't need chemotherapy, whereas someone like me, with a relatively small lump that was removed in a lumpectomy, did.

My blood counts were the highest they had ever been thanks to the horrible Neulasta injection. The white cells had risen from a paltry 3,500 to a magnificent 9,700. The chemo receptionist said: 'Vous êtes une merveille, Madame Kershaw, c'est genial!' My fifth and penultimate chemo passed almost pleasantly. A friend met me at the hospital and we ate banana and walnut cake, shortbread and drank green tea and chatted non-stop until the drugs ran dry.

I chatted with Sus as she put on her protective rubber gloves to plug in my final bag of drugs. She was training for the Nice

Ironman event, comprising a 3.8 km swim, a 130 km bike ride and a full marathon. I said: 'Amazing, you make me feel very lazy by comparison,' to which she retorted: 'Hey, you have run marathons and even on chemo you are running 5 km. All I can say to you is respect.'

I saw my GP and told him I was continuing to run and do yoga and hadn't been sick at all.

He said: 'I have a lot of cancer patients, many of whom have had chemotherapy, and it's very rare to hear any of them talk like this.' He also described the radiotherapy doctor standing in the way of my job in Toronto by insisting on a several week gap between chemo and radiotherapy as 'a miserable bastard,' adding: 'One of my patients told me that she made him laugh once, which is nothing short of a miracle!'

Buoyed by his support, I started working my way up to another plea for speed and clemency at my next appointment with Movie Star but word had clearly reached him already and he got there first.

'Why do you want to speed up the treatment?' he asked as soon as I sat down. When I explained that I had barely worked for three months and had a lucrative job in Toronto in April, he said: 'You look good and you're withstanding the chemotherapy very well. I don't see why you shouldn't go off and do your work.' My weight had gone up to 49 kg, a kilo more than my last weigh-in, and that sealed the deal.

Movie Star's lovely secretary Sylvie faced a battle on the phone to my radiotherapy doctor to ensure that I could start 'les rayons' a week after finishing chemotherapy instead of the normal four or five week gap. She persevered and hung up with a smile, saying: 'You will be prepped for radiotherapy on January 31st, ready to start on February 14th.' Forget chocolates, roses or Champagne, this was the most magnificent Valentine's gift imaginable. I was due to leave on a three week Transatlantic trip just four days after finishing treatment, but I felt no fear, only elation at having my normal life reinstated after so long.

I thought I had encountered all the side effects but there was still one more to come. The menopausal night sweats were something else. I veered between feeling so cold that I was sleeping for the first time ever in sweat pants and a long sleeved T shirt to raging sweats where my head felt like it was trapped inside a boiling kettle. They didn't last long, a matter of minutes, and seemed to occur most often at night, in bed. Occasionally I would turn into a hot, sweaty beetroot while doing an interview or meeting a client but the daytime sweats were thankfully less frequent.

On days when I didn't feel so bad, I'd run gently with the dogs but 5k was now the equivalent of a half marathon in terms of the effort it took. I'd do yoga, go out for lunch and to the movies and when I wasn't up to anything more taxing than sitting on the sofa, I'd be armed with my iPad, BlackBerry, notebook and diary, dealing with emails, blogs, telephone calls, research and general time wasting on technology. Years of working meant I felt guilty not doing something, even if I felt sleepy.

The drugs messed with my mind as well as my body. Regularly, I would lose track in the middle of a conversation, even forgetting the names of great friends. The right words also eluded me. Trying to make myself useful one day, I rang the tile shop to ask if I could exchange the grout we bought for the swimming pool for a darker shade. Checking the words I needed on my iPad, I struggled to think of the word for grout in English! 'Comment dire en Anglais' is not a question I was used to asking in France.

If I didn't write down every little thing, I'd forget where I was going or who I was supposed to be meeting. I left the house one morning and got halfway up the drive before realizing I had absolutely no idea where I was going. Speaking as someone who has always taken a photographic memory for granted, this was worrying. I had to cancel dinner with friends after double booking us and I lost count of the times the girls said to me, 'Mum, we've told you three times already, why aren't you listening?'

I went food shopping one day with Iain, who dropped me at the supermarket and left me there while he went off to get more cement for the pool. When he met me mid-aisle, he mentioned various conversations we'd supposedly had, which I had no recollection of, and then lost the will to live when we reached the cash desk and he saw that I had not weighed any of the vegetables or fruit being squashed by beers and wine at the bottom of the trolley. On another occasion, I managed to leave a huge carton of expensive pool cleaning fluid in my trolley while loading the car with shopping and drive off oblivious before realizing halfway home. I performed a crazy U-turn on our narrow road like a woman possessed and sped back to the store car park only to find that a nasty piece of work had already stolen it.

After three months of chemo, every bone in my body ached, right down to the nail beds underneath my fingernails. But it was important to plan things to do post chemo so that I didn't sit at home moping about how rubbish I felt. I knew there were a lot of people who had suffered far worse through chemo than I was suffering so little excursions here and there became the pattern.

A few hours after my fifth treatment, I was tucking into fish curry and a glass of champagne at our local Indian restaurant. It felt good to be out and not be feeling even slightly nauseous. And the following evening, I wore my vertiginous Gucci boots to walk to a nearby restaurant to meet friends for dinner. I'm not sure what I was trying to prove but it was made worthwhile when my friends remarked on how well I looked and how mad I was wearing boots that high. Those boots had sat in a box for five months so it was high time they saw some action.

And breathe…Don't forget that however interminable, rough and endless the treatment seems, it is temporary and once it's over, you will start to feel and look normal again.

Chapter Eighteen

Woolly Hats Work Wonders

The only upside to having treatment during the colder months was being able to wrap up and wear hats. Layers made me look less thin and a hat made the wig look a little less wiggy. I was relieved I wouldn't have to endure a wig in the summer heat. Hard though it was to physically lug my body around, being out in the elements on a weekend ski trip and guiding myself gently down the slopes as my thighs burned was worth the effort.

Hair or no hair, I had decided I was not going to miss the start of ski season, after all, it would be a great excuse to hide under a big woolly hat.

After a balmy, sunny December and January, we had endured a snowless ski season in the southern Alpes Maritimes, which seemed to signal a relaxing non-skiing trip of spas and bars on our weekend break in Foux d'Allos in the Var, a prospect that Iain, who is always happiest when unclipping his skis at the nearest bar to the slopes, was relishing. Having endured five chemo sessions with just one left, I, on the other hand, was looking forward to some action on the slopes as I was on a 'good' week.

Iain made a huge pot of Thai chicken curry so the girls wouldn't starve as they opted to stay at home rather than join us on the slopes. I filled the fridge with appealing foods instead of

Tupperware containers filled with weird and wonderful recipes from my food plan. I even bought oven chips as a special treat although I felt dreadful about putting them in my shopping basket. After trying Ovaltine with rice milk, Liv gagged before declaring that she'd rather give it up altogether than try another cup of hot chocolate Karen style so it was only fair that they had a weekend off my food plan products.

I left strict instructions on feeding and walking the dogs, and the girls were more excited about having the house to themselves than we were about going away. They were planning to languish in PJs, unwashed, snacking on pizza and chocolate and watching Celebrity Big Brother until we arrived back home.

I was looking forward to seeing how I would fare on the slopes for an entire weekend but lugging my skis and poles from the car park in the centre of town to the lift a mere 100 metres away was hard enough. The first run, a red, was painful on my calves and thighs, which began to burn like crazy.

'Are you ok?' Iain asked at the bottom.

'Yes,' I lied. He only needed the tiniest incentive to quit for a large glass of red in front of a roaring fire at a bar. As we ate pizza and drank wine at lunchtime, he confessed that if he was with his friends, he wouldn't even venture out of the restaurant again until closing time. But he was with me. And I wanted to ski.

By the end of the third run, the burning sensation in my legs had subsided and despite the grey day and not altogether brilliant conditions, I felt free, normal and alive, even though the super duper high factor sun cream on my face had turned me blue and made me look like a corpse. As if I needed any help on that score. Two hours later, lying in a scented bath back at the hotel, I felt the lovely physical tiredness of exercise rather than the interminable lethargic exhaustion caused by drugs.

Meanwhile, there was an earthquake in the Italian region of Liguria which measured 5.3 on the Richter scale and the tremors were felt as far afield as the Var, the Alpes Maritimes and Grasse. Liv rang to say that her school building was shaking so much that a projector had fallen to the floor and smashed, causing widespread panic among the students. Sensibly, they evacuated the Lycée while poor Issy, who was at the college building, was forced to continue playing ping pong in the gym! French teachers don't get fazed by much. I wanted to laugh but given that I was 100 km away from my babies while they endure a minor earthquake, it would have made me a very bad momma indeed.

We awoke on Saturday morning to light blizzards which freshened up conditions beautifully after six weeks of no white stuff. While the rest of our ski party was punching the air with delight, Iain was quietly gutted at the prospect of half a metre of fresh powder. Some of the funnier comments I heard muttered behind me were: 'I feel like I've just hiked up the Eiger with a Mini on my back,' 'Welcome to Hell,' 'My thighs feel like they have been smashed with giant mallets,' and on spotting the bodies of powder virgins strewn across the piste below us, he quipped: 'It's like a scene from Casualty.'

We spent the day enjoying the most challenging skiing I'd experienced in 12 months on un-groomed red runs and off piste powder with virtually no visibility due to continuous snow and low cloud. It was amazing and although I was shattered by late afternoon, the hammam and steam room at the hotel restored me. I did get a few strange looks for wearing the black nylon swimming hat I had hastily picked up from Decathlon. I was relieved I had decided against baldly striding into the spa when I spotted the five hot young snowboarders in the steam room. It was a choice between looking a bit mad in a swimming cap or not using the spa through embarrassment and I plumped for the former.

I went off-piste on the food plan too. There is no such thing as gluten free, sugar free, meat free, dairy free fare in an Alpine ski resort. It's fondue, raclette, pizza, pasta and hearty meat stews all the way so I started each day with an almond croissant and a latte. A couple of goats' cheese salads were thrown in alongside a couple of very cheesy pizzas.

Being away from home took my mind off the misery of treatment, as did the return journey, which was an eventful three and a half hour drive through blizzards along snow packed passes and narrow cols with sheer drops. The satellite navigation system in the car inexplicably bypassed snow-free Castellane to take us on a climb through medieval villages at the top of the world which would have been gloriously picturesque in the summer but in failing light and snow storms was terrifying.

As Iain braked to put the car into four wheel drive mode, we started slipping backwards towards a snowy ditch. The signal on our phones went kaput and despite gentle acceleration, the car was slipping backwards off the road towards a snow filled field in the middle of nowhere. Iain had to get out and wrestle to get the snow socks onto the front tyres before we finally managed to edge the car back on the road and creep along the scariest pass of all, some 1000 metres high in thick blizzards, on skating rink style roads with not a snow plough in sight.

As my blunt-talking American friend Susie said afterwards: 'Can you imagine going through those operations, chemo and losing your hair only to bite the dust skidding off a snowy cliff face?'

Heavy snowfall meant our road was closed and most side roads nearby were impassable. School was also closed and effectively we were snowed in with no transport. But after such a terrifying journey, I felt a little bit invincible and decided it was time to get rid of the annoying last vestiges of what passed for hair on my head once and for all.

I told Iain: 'I think I'm going to get you to shave my head. I look ridiculous with all this old lady bum fluff. I look like nan from The Catherine Tate Show. At least I might look a little less old if I was completely bald. I'll be able to see when my hair starts growing back. And I won't have to faff about with pathetic pea-sized amounts of shampoo anymore.'

He looked alarmed. 'I don't want you to get rid of it. It's nice to see you with a little bit of hair, Tufty. I'm quite attached to those flossy bits. But if you really want to do it, I will shave it off for you.'

After carrying my skis as well as his own to and from the car all weekend and making numerous trips from our hotel room to the car to fetch things I'd forgotten, he had now offered to shave my head. This was love.

All four of us crammed into the bathroom and Iain rubbed shaving cream all over my scalp. The girls were agog and didn't want to miss out on this spectacle. Finally, I had stopped feeling so emotional about my hair. It felt strangely empowering to be getting rid of the bum fluff after many weeks of comb-overs, hair clogging the plughole and unpleasant shedding all over the floor and bed. The 10% of straggly mess that was left on my head bore no resemblance to the long glossy hair I had before cancer so it was easy not to get upset.

Issy sat on the loo seat Googling bald actresses after I told her that Cameron Diaz, Cynthia Nixon and Natalie Portman had all shaved their heads for acting roles.

The iPad came in handy every time there was a power cut too. Issy would jump into position holding the screen near my head to shine some light as Iain continued to shave with a Bic razor. Magnanimous to the last, after skimming through the final strands, he donated his Burberry after shave balm to me, saying: 'You need this more than I do.'

Looking in the mirror afterwards, it struck me how much more like me I looked. The girls stared at my head and Issy piped up: 'Actually mum, you do look a lot better now with your head shaved.' Liv nodded her approval and Iain found himself agreeing. The unkempt pensioner was gone. I was no longer Catherine Tate's nan, more Natalie Portman's mum.

And breathe…Indulge yourself and book a weekend away. It's impossible to travel much during treatment but you'd be amazed at the healing power of a 48 hour escape to a hotel and a change of scenery.

Chapter Nineteen

Radio Gaga

At the end of chemotherapy, I felt emotion as well as huge relief about saying goodbye to my team. I was dehydrated (you need to drink around three litres of water a day at this stage), but the miracle Neulasta jabs had worked their magic and kept my blood counts within normal range. I had cleared the hardest of hurdles and I was finally on the home strait. So why did I feel so tearful?

At the end of January, just a week before my final chemotherapy treatment, I met my radiotherapy doctor who replaced the grump I was supposed to get. He was charming and kind and took his time explaining exactly what would happen over the following few weeks. He showed me a diagram of the lymph node 'ladder'. My one bad lymph node with the small carcinoma had been on a chain of nodes which ran from under my right arm up to my shoulder and down my sternum so it was vital to radiate the whole of this chain in case any other rogue cells had developed.

As with all the treatment, the risks were outlined, including an increased chance of developing cancer in the future, but one major fact I had learned was the importance of making decisions based on the here and now, not what could happen further down the line.

After months of the usual chemo routine, early February saw a flurry of activity with seven appointments in the space of a week to finish off the chemo and start the radiotherapy. A normal patient would have had five to six weeks of no treatment at all to regain strength, breathe a little more easily and set themselves up for the next phase. I had six days. It was impossible to make plans or lead anything like a normal life with a diary that was packed with hospital visits rather than exciting assignments but at least the end of treatment was now in sight. Knowing how close I was to the finish line made everything worthwhile.

I weighed in at 51 kg for my final pre-chemo rendezvous with Movie Star, which was great news. He remarked that I was dehydrated, adding: 'It's very common at this stage in chemo. I can see the lines around your eyes, have you noticed them?'

I didn't like to say I'd noticed them about five years ago! Sadly, this was one thing I couldn't blame the chemo for. (And I have to say the French skincare brand Absolution performed miracles on them post treatment).

Movie Star said I would look and feel completely normal again in two months, which seemed impossible to believe. Well, I would still be a skinhead, so not quite normal looking. He also warned that Tamoxifen had side effects similar to the pill including a higher risk of thrombosis, dry skin, hot flushes and mood swings. I was experiencing blurred vision and my eyes watered a lot as a result of the chemotherapy. But I was encouraged by an email from Isabella, who told me that since starting Tamoxifen after her mastectomy, she'd had no adverse side effects, mood swings, flushes or depression. She wanted to reassure me that it was not as bad as we both feared.

At the end of my consultation, I gave Movie Star a thank you card and he seemed touched. A man of few words, he showed it to his secretary and wished me 'bon continuation.'

It was a relief to collect my blood results and see that they were within normal range ready for my final chemotherapy AT LAST. Four months had felt like four years. Every day I'd had to push myself towards a goal. When I had down days full of pain, fatigue and sheer misery, I forced myself to remember that on February 7th 2012, five months after diagnosis, the most gruelling part of my treatment would be finished.

Despite all the horrible things chemo wrought on my body, I was feeling very emotional about my last treatment. I had become attached to my chemo team, especially Dr Hoch and Sus. Their brilliance, kindness and support had gone a long way to making me feel human again, they had saved my life and they had become my allies. I knew I would miss them but I was sure they would understand when I said I never wanted to see them again!

Milly came to my last chemo and we laughed and chatted our way through the session. The old lady opposite almost had a fit when I whipped off my wig to show Milly my new look shiny, smooth bald head. She then proceeded to choke on her coffee when Milly produced a bottle of Champagne and asked Sus if we could drink it. Sus did her best to look stern as she told us that no, we were not allowed to uncork it on the ward, so as soon as I was unhooked from the IV line, we hotfooted it back to the car and knocked back plastic glasses full of celebration bubbles in the underground car park like a couple of teenagers.

Driving home, the sun was shining so we stopped off for a late celebratory lunch in Valbonne. It was like someone had let me out of a dark room into sunlight. I felt elated. As the hours passed, I had no nausea and just a little fatigue. I seemed to be proof that going into chemotherapy well informed, following a clean diet and on the right supplements, minerals and vitamins could set your body up for withstanding even the most horrific side effects quite well.

One of these was my bleeding hands. The first time it happened was as I packed groceries into carrier bags at the supermarket. I lightly brushed the top of my hand across the bag handle and suddenly there was blood everywhere. My skin had become so delicate and paper thin from the Taxotere that it was flaking off like extreme sunburn and exploding in little blood blisters.

I had become addicted to reading cancer blogs in a bid to second guess everything that would be happening to me and I stumbled across one written by Karen George in Arizona, snappily titled Fighting-breast-cancer.com. Repeatedly told not to worry about a lump she found in her breast, it wasn't until she developed a persistent hacking cough several months later that she was finally given a scan. What had started off as breast cancer had by then spread to her spinal cord, her lungs and rib cage. The cancer cells lit up her body like a fairground in the scan, she said. She was Stage IV thanks to an incompetent initial diagnosis of a harmless cyst.

Somehow she kept an amusing, witty and sometimes bleak blog about her fight, never once losing her sense of humour and making readers like me laugh out loud, albeit through a veil of tears. When her entries stopped abruptly one day, I searched high and low on the net looking for some trace of Karen and eventually stumbled on a comment from her husband Michael telling her readers that she had lost her fight three years after diagnosis at the age of 33.

When everyone around you is full of bonhomie and reassuring murmurs of how fine you're going to be (often to make themselves feel better because the alternative is too painful too consider), a story like Karen's is a grim reminder that you should always trust your instincts, no matter what any doctor might tell you.

My modus operandi was to make myself as well informed as possible and fill my body with the good stuff that might, just might, play a part in killing off the bad guys. As a mental exercise, it also worked on the level that you felt like you were doing something good and useful for yourself. So adding fresh herbs from the garden to my cooking and buying much of my produce at the farmer's market every Monday morning, where the vegetables, fruit, fish, rotisserie chickens, cheeses, girolles and oyster mushrooms are locally raised or sourced and have seen very little in the way of preservatives or pesticides, gave me an active role in managing my health and my illness.

Equally important was my desire to keep exercising, despite everyone telling me to slow down and rest. I went running in minus 4 degrees one February morning, just to prove I could still do it. I could do it but it was hard and a pretty stupid thing to do. I lasted half an hour but that was 15 minutes too long in freezing winds with my bald head and trusty cashmere beanie. Heading uphill along an almost vertical winding lane beat me but it would beat me before cancer too so I was quietly pleased with myself.

Tattoo day arrived and I went for a scan to pinpoint exactly where the radiotherapy needed to be directed. I took off my jumper and bra and lay on a mobile bed with my arms raised above my head and my head tilted to the left, perfectly still. The bed slowly moved into the scanner and my upper half was scanned while the two radiographers mapped out the dots – seven in total – and marked them with pen using the laser aperture while measuring the co-ordinates. I was marked from the top of my right breastbone down across the right breast and nipple.

Then I was tattooed with a needle and black dye. X marked the spot, well, seven spots. The tattoos were only semi-permanent which was just as well because if I wanted tattoos I wouldn't go for black crosses!

Afterwards I looked like I'd been scratching around up the chimney but the consultant radiologist told me that after a shower, I'd be left with just little black dots rather than big fat black blobs.

The scene was set for three minute blasts each weekday for six and a half weeks, with 25 sessions on the lymph node area and the final eight sessions on my breast. The lymph nodes needed more treatment because the cancer had started moving whereas the breast lump was in situ.

The latest set of side effects included exceptionally dry skin, sunburn-style redness and tiredness, although the radiologist assured me it would be nothing like the fatigue I'd felt during chemo. I was warned not to use perfume or perfumed soap, deodorant or other scented body products, as well as nothing containing alcohol (usually I drink that rather than rub it on my body!) Underwired bras or anything trimmed with lace was banned in favour of soft cotton. The sun was to be avoided at all costs on the right side of my upper body for a year , which meant that at least my wrinkles would be getting a breather.

I should have been feeling upbeat about heading into the third stage, after all it wasn't going to be anywhere as near as brutal as what I had already endured. But I didn't have the energy to feel anything other than worn out. Refusing to admit defeat, I agreed to a day ski trip with friends and the following day, although my legs ached like I had walked barefoot up Everest, in my head, I had chalked up another small victory.

And breathe…Try and do half an hour of exercise or activity a day, whether it's walking the dog, playing tennis, swimming, a gentle jog around the block or some gentle yoga.

Chapter Twenty

All Zapped Out

The fatigue that comes with cancer treatment is quite something. I felt 120 years old (I looked it too), making polite and sparkling dinner party conversation was beyond me and the prospect of lying down for radiotherapy every day was appealing, even if the sunburn and itchiness caused by the rays was not. Avoiding perfumed beauty products was good advice as they made my skin even more irritable.

By mid-February, five months since diagnosis, I was counting the days for the effects of chemo to leave my system. It can take your body up to a year to recover but after a week, the bitter metallic taste was already gone and the general tiredness and malaise was lessening. However, I felt totally washed out. My entire body was at its lowest ebb and still I couldn't say no. I took Liv to our local ski resort and we skied in minus 15 degrees, which wasn't pleasant but I didn't want to let her down. Not that she would have minded. I minded. We stayed in the mountains for a couple of hours after which we were both ready to head home, defrosting our feet and hands on the journey back with the car heater up full blast.

Going out to dinner has always been one of my favourite things but it had become a huge effort. We were invited over to a friend's house for supper and everyone was standing up drinking Champagne and chatting by the roaring log fire. I could see the sofa winking at me but for some reason I didn't suggest sitting down until Fiona saw how tired I looked and insisted. At dinner, I felt glazed and was unusually quiet. I lasted until just before 1am but it caused a total wipeout the following day.

It was a stark realization to find that the way I was feeling was the reason for building in several weeks' recovery from chemo before starting radiotherapy. I was exhausted. My gap, after relentlessly lobbying my team, of six days in order to fit in the Toronto trip ahead of LA and Palm Springs had felt perfectly doable until this moment.

Depression is common among cancer sufferers but I never got depressed. That's not to say I didn't feel down sometimes or fed up with the general boring daily grind of treatment and nausea (luckily it was just a feeling and not actual sickness, which I am eternally grateful for). I really missed getting out of bed with a spring in my step, ready for the day ahead. At times, it was more of an old lady stagger than a spring. I felt weak and out of sorts. I missed brushing my hair. It was an effort to brush my teeth. But not once did I feel the grip of such despair that I wanted to give up.

In Karen's blog, which her husband started updating following her death in August 2008, she says: 'With cancer you have to be a fighter. I cannot be accepting when cancer tells me no. Each chemo is another round in the ring with cancer. Each scan is a sparring match. I get weary; sometimes I get knocked down. But I always get my tired, puffy, bruised body back up and fight some more.' This is exactly what it's like. But to do this, you have to believe you are going to win, even if that feels like a leap of faith.

Believing in myself was one thing but I had no control over how everyone around me dealt with my cancer. Liv and Issy were old enough to understand the gravity of my illness but young enough to feel horribly vulnerable and sick with fear at what was happening to their hitherto sporty, carefree, young-ish, fit and healthy mum.

In the early days after diagnosis, I asked them to come to me with their fears, worries and questions about cancer and what it might do to me and what my treatment would be like. Taking myself out of the equation, I was interested in the psychology of how children, teenagers in particular, cope with a life threatening illness so I did what I'm good at and interviewed them about it. Our chat was revealing. They kept their questions and fears to themselves and didn't even discuss it with each other, which surprised me.

Liv told me: 'The night you told us you had cancer, I thought, 'That's it, you are going to die.' It didn't help that two years earlier your friend Lisa had died of cancer. Sometimes I thought maybe I had done something that had triggered it off in you. And I would think, 'Maybe if we hadn't had that argument, Mum might not have got cancer.'

Issy nodded, adding: 'We didn't like talking about it. I never spoke about it to Dad. I was scared I might make him cry and I don't like to see Dad cry. I was really angry. You didn't do anything bad, you didn't over-drink or smoke, you were so healthy. You do lots of sport and yoga so I didn't understand why it had to happen to you out of all the people it could happen to.' I didn't understand this either but there is no point dwelling on why me...it's more a case of well, it gets one in three, so why not me?

My oncologist friend Dr Sarah in the UK said: 'I wish I could get you to London to talk to some of my cancer patients. Keeping positive and upbeat is so important; it makes a real difference to your progress.'

On Valentine's Day, I arrived for my first radiotherapy session on a machine called Artemis, named after the goddess of hunting and the wilderness. An apt name considering this Artemis was hunting down and burning any remaining cancer cells. I met my two lovely female radiologists who would be my companions for the next 32 sessions and they could not have been kinder.

'The hardest part of this treatment will be driving here and back every day,' one of them told me in French, which was music to my ears.

I stripped to the waist and lay next to the state of the art Artemis, which lined up each of my seven tattoos before painlessly zapping each one. At one point, as I stared into the glass screen above my head with my arms raised, I felt just like James Bond in the scene where Goldfinger is lasering him. The red line ran down across my right breast and I could see the coordinates in the glass reflection exactly meeting at the point of the tattoo, which was highlighted in red marker pen. After a series of beeps, buzzes and clicks, the most simple, pain-free part of treatment so far was over.

They had to slot me into holes in the schedule for the first two weeks just to get started as my treatment plan had been speeded up, but for the final month I was given a teatime slot each day, which was ideal for getting me out of cooking supper.

The best part about radiotherapy was the chance to lie down in a quiet room every day. On each visit I got used to seeing the same familiar faces of other patients…the lady with the baseball cap, defiantly refusing to wear a wig, a couple of older ladies wearing wigs and a younger one in a bandana. There was an unspoken camaraderie among us all. We smiled at each other and said bonjour and au revoir but we didn't chat.

To break the monotony of five trips a week to the Tzanck, I invented my own version of Beat The Clock. Getting out of the car park in less than 30 minutes per visit was nigh on impossible but the incentive was the first 30 minutes parking was free, and after that it was a euro an hour. Small stakes but it made my daily visits a bit more interesting. The trick was to get there just five minutes before my time slot and after being blasted, hurriedly put my clothes on and hurtle to the car park machine in the corridor to validate my ticket. Given that treatment lasted a total of 15 to 20 minutes by the time each spot had been zapped, it was always a close run thing.

Some days were more competitive than others, depending on my mood and energy levels, and I would plan my wardrobe in advance, choosing flip flops and a dress to make getting dressed a few valuable seconds quicker. On the jeans, shirt and Converse days, I really had my work cut out. My best time was 26 minutes and this was on a Converse day. I had to pay six times in total, meaning there were 26 days when I beat the clock.

To begin with, the soreness wasn't too bad. I had the perpetual feeling that I had pulled a muscle across my right shoulder blade. It was red, inflamed and itchy. My biggest problem was that my eyes watered constantly. I had about eight eyebrow hairs left on each side and barely any eyelashes and it seemed to be the lack of protection from the elements that was causing my constant weepiness. It meant that the myriad pairs of sunglasses I had accumulated were finally getting plenty of wear but there were times when my constantly weeping eyes could be incredibly embarrassing.

I had a meeting with an artist in Mougins with a view to writing a piece on him but from the moment I arrived at his studio, my eyes streamed so much that I had to pretend I had a violent cold. It was embarrassing sitting there weeping while he showed me his canvases. The discoloration under my fingernails had also deepened to a rancid dark yellow/green, giving the impression that I must be a 100 a day smoker, so the threat of losing them was back again.

But at least the embarrassment of being bald had disappeared. It was only a problem when people unexpectedly spotted me without my wig. Our pool tiler put his head round the door one morning and reeled from the vision of me sitting at my PC as bald as a baby's backside. And sharing a takeaway curry one evening, my friends didn't know where to look when I whipped off my wig after one asked me if I needed to shave my head much. Their faces were a picture and the next morning I received a text from one saying: 'Great seeing you last night, with or without the Star Trek look! You are an inspiration.'

In the spirit of feeling braver, I decided I didn't want to wake up any longer to be greeted by the sight of two wigs on their stands on the bedroom fireplace. It was the most depressing sight to start my day with and a constant reminder of cancer so I hid them in my wardrobe and in their place, I displayed lots of framed photographs of the girls when they were little, Iain and I on our wedding day in Mauritius and other memories that had been tucked in a box and forgotten about.

Two weeks into radiotherapy and three weeks post chemo at the beginning of March, I was finally feeling stronger. My legs ached so running was still on hold more often than not but my hacking cough had gone and the pain under my fingernails, which had been excruciating, had almost disappeared. Two friends who hadn't seen me since December commented on how much better

I was looking so the couple of kilos I'd put on seemed to make up for what I lacked in hair and general glamour.

My physio continued to be painful but at an appointment with Clooney, he told me to push my right arm to the limit to get it properly mobile again so I booked tennis and did some strenuous arm stretches in yoga which hurt but released some of the build-up of tension.

My discoloured fingernails were the result of dystrophy caused by the drugs and would not fall off, he assured me, but would grow out as the nail grew. Ditto my blurred vision, also drug induced, would improve along with the constantly weeping eyes.

As I left, Clooney said: 'It's good to see you again.' The last time I was in his office the previous autumn, I left in tears after being told that the cancer had invaded a lymph node and I needed another operation and chemotherapy. This time, my exit was a happy one.

With chemo now over, Simone and I had a Skype call to talk through my food plan. I scored five out of 10 in the pee test, which she declared as nothing short of miraculous. It was not unusual to score one or two out of 10 at this stage of treatment so to be at 50% was amazing. I was still dehydrated, acidic and one of my liver markers was struggling, plus the parasite was partying for all it was worth but my vitamin and mineral levels were good, my other liver marker was tip top and my urinary tract looked good too.

The plan was to maintain everything until the end of radiotherapy, and then go for a major detox to rid my system of any remaining chemo or radio. Simone was designing a travel pack for my trips in April and she told me: 'Your results are fab, I'm super proud of you for sticking to the plan.' It was a fatal error to tell me how well I'd done because it just made me want to fall off the wagon into a vat of chocolate. We talked cheating (I couldn't help being honest with her, it was like being a Catholic at confession) and she confessed to a weakness for Haagen Dazs. I celebrated by drinking two glasses of bubbly and eating a crème brulée.

In the interests of complete honesty, there were two other conditions to add to my burgeoning list of side effects....piles and flatulence. I decided to share a funny story with Faye during our yoga session and we spent 15 minutes in hysterical laughter on the floor as I talked about the elegant Singaporean lady in my pilates class back in London who used to sit behind me each week and ruffle my hair whenever her wind went free in a certain position. This lady never acknowledged her little problem, meaning that the instructor and I had to avoid eye contact for the rest of the session as we stifled our childish giggles. Now that lady was me!

As for the piles, let's just say that me and Germoloids were becoming intimately acquainted despite the fact that I was eating more fruit and vegetables than a pregnant rabbit.

And breathe….Be honest about how you're feeling and stop trying to protect everyone around you. You are No.1 for a while and nobody will mind if you put yourself first. As a female and a mum, this is a tough nut to crack!

Chapter Twenty One

The Guinea Wig

I was slowly becoming more relaxed about my close family seeing me without hair but there were limits to my courage. And that was okay. As someone who has always tried to push myself beyond my comfort zone, I was starting to realise that sometimes it was just fine to stay within it too.

Why do people always knock on the door just as I've taken my wig off? One of our neighbours popped in for a coffee so I had to hurriedly slap it back on as he came through the door. I looked like Derek Jacobi in Cadfael although he was too polite to say anything.

I had been planning to go shopping, lunching and mooching in Cannes without my wig just to see if it was possible to wander around and blend in while looking like an anaemic boiled egg but when it came down to it, I wimped out. I wanted to be brave enough to stick two fingers up at anyone who stared at me in the street and give a happy high five to strangers who were confident enough to look me in the eye, I really did. But after so many months of looking and feeling different, what I wanted most of all was to conform, not defiantly stand out from the crowd. And going bald in rue d'Antibes - Cannes' version of Bond Street - would not go unnoticed.

It was easier to be a rebel in the safety of my own four walls. Milly came over for lunch and we sat on the terrace with my wig casually perched between our mugs of camomile tea on the table. It spent more time on work surfaces and coffee tables than on my head at home, although I made sure it was always close enough to hand to put on as soon as Issy walked in through the door after school.

'I really wish I had my camera,' said Milly, gesturing to the carelessly discarded heap of hair in front of us, 'that would make such a great photo.' The photo opportunity did not pass unnoticed by Iain, who placed some lettuce leaves next to it and took a photo with his phone before emailing it to a few of his mates for a very politically incorrect laugh. One friend texted back to say he had been crying with laughter at the picture, while his wife thought it was in very poor taste indeed.

'She just sent a message back to me branding us both evil,' said Iain, his shoulders shaking with laughter. 'Sorry, but it looks like a guinea pig when you leave it lying around like that.'

I thought it was rather funny, too, and from then on, it became known as the guinea wig. If I didn't know better, I would also be fooled by this amazing doppelganger for a small furry animal.

It seemed like the perfect solution to Issy's constant request for a guinea pig. When she was tiny, she loved to collect the dead mice brought home by our cats and would beg to keep them in an old cereal carton in her room. I suppose the idea of a small furry pet that doesn't struggle to get away from you is quite appealing when you are two years old. A guinea wig would be a cheap, hygienic alternative.

I was feeling more upbeat and in the mood for visitors so Iain arranged for my brother-in-law Gary and his husband Phil to come over and stay, along with my sister-in-law Lisa. We spent five days laughing, relaxing by the newly finished pool, lunching in San Remo and eating delicious food and drinking lovely wine. To say I fell off the wagon was putting it mildly. The wagon had completely derailed.

I decided to go bareheaded at home. It was a big thing to do outside the company of immediate close family, especially as I had no eyebrows or lashes. I took off my wig after we arrived home from the airport and Gary and Phil came over one at a time to hug me and kiss the top of my shiny head. Then Gary made me watch an old Catherine Tate sketch on YouTube and dubbed me Derek Faye, her closet gay bald creation. Any fears I had of him going soft were unfounded.

I was starting to feel so much better, almost normal, and it threw into sharp focus just how rubbish I had felt for the previous couple of months. Being able to get out of bed without feeling breathless was a wonderful thing. As my strength slowly returned, I started playing tennis again after a two month break, just a set at a time, and it was a relief to find I didn't have to go home and lie down for the rest of the day to recover.

I started thinking about training for the Piste to Plage cycle challenge that I had signed up for. Organised by friends, it was an epic 440 km bike ride for four days from the French Alps to the French Riviera to raise money for Help For Heroes. The final day's ride was to take place on September 15th, the first anniversary of my cancer diagnosis, and it seemed like a fitting way of celebrating this very special day as well as giving me a focus for training and regaining my fitness again. But until house to top of drive got easier, Piste to Plage training would have to wait.

At this point, although I looked like the living dead, in my head at least, my standards hadn't slipped too much. I still read Vogue and Grazia in bed, checking out who was on the frow at Paris and London Fashion Weeks, mulling over Spring/Summer looks and wondering which ones would work best with a bald head. Anything high-necked, lace or colour blocked seemed to be the way forward.

Other reading matter included the efficacy of Yun Zhi (Coriolus Versicolor), a particular kind of mushroom, on survival in cancer patients in a scientific report carried out by the School of Public Health and Primary Care at the Chinese University of Hong Kong and the Prince of Wales Hospital, Hong Kong.

'The findings show that Yun Zhi results in a significant survival advantage compared with standard conventional anti-cancer treatment alone,' it read. 'Of patients randomized to Yun Zhi, there was a 9% absolute reduction in five year mortality, resulting in one additional patient alive for every 11 patients treated. In patients with breast cancer, gastric cancer or colorectal cancer treated with chemotherapy, the effects of the combination of Yun Zhi preparation on the overall five year survival rate was more evident, but not in oesophageal cancer and nasopharyngeal carcinoma. However, subgroup analysis could not conclude which type of anti-cancer treatment may maximize the benefit from Yun Zhi.

'This meta-analysis has provided strong evidence that Yun Zhi would have survival benefit in cancer patients, particularly in carcinoma of breast, gastric and colorectal. Nevertheless, the findings highlight the need for further evidence from prospective studies of outcome to guide future potential modifications of treatment regimes.'

I put mushrooms on my shopping list. At times I felt as if cancer was part of my aura. You know how when you want to get pregnant, it seems like pregnant women are everywhere? I felt like cancer was all around me. I interviewed the singer Anastacia and she talked about how positivity got her through her breast cancer battle nine years earlier. It was a struggle to bite my tongue and not tell her my story. Then I received a press release about Five, a collection of five short films by directors including Jennifer Aniston, Demi Moore and Alicia Keys, exploring the impact of breast cancer on people's lives.

Halfway through radiotherapy, I got a chance to travel to London, albeit for the saddest of reasons, to say goodbye to Kitty, my lovely, feisty 95-year-old nan, who was dying. She had stopped eating and had lost all interest in life. The manager at her residential care home had recently discussed an end of life care plan with my mum which meant no resuscitation if she had a heart attack, no feeding tubes, just bed rest and palliative care. She knew nothing of my illness and it was easy to conceal it from her as she had been suffering with Alzheimer's disease for several years and I lived 1,000 miles away so I didn't get to see her very often.

Issy made a beautiful collage of photographs for me to pin up at her bedside and looking at them was a reminder that up until her late 80s, Kitty was full of fun and vitality, the life and soul of the party. She spent her 90th birthday at my house, surrounded by family and friends, dancing around the kitchen to Frank Sinatra wearing a pink stetson while the kids raced up and down the garden in the wheelchair that she hated to use.

Seeing my proud, fastidious, stylish nan lying in bed, her thin wasted legs grotesquely twisted to one side with a pillow beneath her knees to relieve pressure, her face gaunt, hair mussed up from lying in one position on the pillow, eyes closed and mouth half open was a terrible sight. She had deteriorated greatly since I had last seen her three months earlier.

It took 45 minutes to feed her some soup, mashed potato and ice cream and she was barely conscious for the two hours mum and I stayed with her although I held her hand and occasionally she would squeeze it. As we got up to leave, I kissed her forehead and told her I loved her. It meant the world to me when she said: 'I love you too, darling.' I left in tears. I saw her once more before she died in May 2012.

Watching Nan slip away during her last few months taught me a lot about death and the blind fear we associate with dying. She was in a lot of discomfort towards the end that even the high dose painkillers couldn't control. It seems to me that there are good deaths and there are bad deaths. A good death is going to bed one night and not waking up. Ideally, when you are old and have had at least three score years and 10. A bad death is being in pain, suffering, being out of control or perhaps worst of all, dying alone. Those are the things I am fearful of, not death itself, because I have packed so much into my life already that, although I'd really like to stick around, I feel quite lucky. Death is not to be feared; it's the journey we might endure on the way that is far more terrifying.

And breathe…Some days are better than others. There's no shame in having a good cry sometimes. Let it out.

Chapter Twenty Two

Celebrating Stubble

Who knew I would feel like throwing a party when the first signs of stubble appeared on my legs? Amazing what you miss when it's gone. I wasn't quite so pleased to discover the hairs starting to sprout on my chin! As for the sunburn from 33 sessions of daily radiotherapy, aloe gel helped to heal the redness and was the only product I found that was gentle enough not to sting like hell.

I went for my first run in five weeks. It was 4 km on the flat and it hurt. I did interval training on the way out - for that, read a walk every five minutes - and one straight run all the way home. On the way back, the pesky wind picked up and my wig started blowing. The only thing worse than being whistled at by the local road works team is being stared at like you're some kind of freak with hair standing bolt upright to attention and attractive wig netting on full view. I put my head down like a raging bull in full charge, which seemed to keep most of the hair in place and made me look like the runner I once was. By the time I got back, I'd been out for 40 minutes and just knowing I had done it was an achievement.

The weather was warming up nicely considering it was early March but for the first time I couldn't take advantage of the first temperate rays of early spring. I was over halfway through radiotherapy and had sores on my back which bled from time to time and my chest was starting to discolour as I had been warned it might. Impressive orange scorch marks covered most of my right side and made me look like an extra from The Only Way is Essex, with a Tango-style burn under my right arm. Direct sunlight was strictly off limits for my poor radiated body so when I sat outside without my wig, I had to wrap up in layers as well as a panama hat and a linen scarf, looking like a dead ringer for Quentin Crisp.

However, I was allowed to get my legs out and I was rubbing high factor sunscreen on them when I noticed a roughness to my usually smooth shins. It was the first sign of stubble growing back. We all cheered....after four months, my body hair had decided to make a comeback (although I was still to find out just how torturously long it would take to grow back on my head.) I also noticed a line of fine hairs just above both ears - the first place I lost my hair - and felt like crying with joy. Then I noticed that they were silvery white! Relief that it was actually going to grow back was tempered by fury that it was coming back grey. The blonde downy hairs on my face and chin were also returning and growing back far thicker than expected, which was not so great either. Iain thought it was amusing to offer me laser hair removal for my birthday. I grouchily declined.

Issy was coming round to her bald mummy finally. She was insisting less and less on me wearing the wig when she was around and was elated at the sight of new growth on my head. As she inspected my scalp she said: 'I'm sure it's horrible being bald mummy but at least you don't have that really annoying thing of your hair tickling you on your back all the time like I do.' I'd never looked at it like that before.

Out for lunch, I spotted a very stylish waitress with a shaved head, neat little sideburns and a slightly longer quiff on top. She was so cool, I thought about taking a sneaky pic on my phone to show my hairdresser for when I had anything to cut but fearing she might mistake me for a lesbian stalker, I decided against it.

Sarah arrived from London for a surprise weekend visit, which was a tonic. We enjoyed a weekend of banned substances - Champagne and coffee – and ate wonderful food which I could taste properly and talked non-stop until Sunday morning when she had to return home. She cried as we said goodbye at the airport, but this time they were tears of happiness, as she told me how much better I looked this time compared to her last visit three months earlier.

There was just one more intervention to go, the removal of the IV drugs line in my chest. After an antiseptic shower with stinky red Betadine, I drove myself to hospital for a rendezvous with Clooney. The procedure took ten minutes. After wheeling me into my usual operating theatre, he swabbed me with Betadine again, covered me with a medical sheet so I couldn't see what was going on (thank God for that) and injected the local anaesthetic, which was the most painful part. He cut through my flesh, opening up a small area on the left side of my chest. The strangest thing was being able to feel him rooting around inside my chest for the IV line and pulling it out without actually feeling any pain.

As he stitched me up, the medical thread pulled jerkily across my chest as the needle went in and out but it was only mild discomfort and was over very quickly. Considering it was the most minor procedure, it left the nastiest, most obvious scar out of all three ops and temporarily made sleeping a nightmare. Unable to lie on my right side because of the burns, now I couldn't lie on my left side or my front.

But at least the first phase of radiotherapy was over. The team took fresh images and zapped my right breast for the first of eight treatments in the final phase, which gave my existing red raw bits a chance to start healing now they had been fully roasted. I could hardly believe it was almost over.

Casting my mind back to the previous autumn, I vividly remembered thinking: 'Well, that's my first chemotherapy out of the way, only five more to go.' Then: 'Ok, now just six weeks of radiotherapy to get through.' Now I could allow myself to think: 'That bottle of Ruinart is going to taste beautiful next Monday evening.' It was a weird feeling knowing that pretty soon, the daily hospital journeys, burns, red dots and chats with the kind radiographers would be history.

The last day of treatment dawned. Liv wanted to come with me. When we arrived in the cosy waiting room, I noticed a couple I hadn't seen before. In their late 60s, they sat together nervously holding hands and I welled up thinking about how frightened they must be at the start of their journey. I went into the changing room to get undressed and as I waited to be called in, I heard the radiographer wishing the lady who was always just before me 'plein de bonnes choses' which means good luck. She was on her last treatment too, and again, I felt tears pricking my eyes at the thought of someone else being through their nightmare and able to start a new chapter.

When I came back to get dressed after being zapped, having also been wished 'plein de bonnes choses', I could hear the radiographer explaining the process to one half of the new couple. It was the husband, who had been squeezing his worried wife's hand just before I went in. She was sitting patiently in the waiting room. I smiled and she smiled back although her face was furrowed with worry.

My radiotherapy doctor checked me over, declared me 'impeccable' after checking my scars and dots, and told me to book an appointment for three months' time with my GP. He also said I had a one in four chance of my periods returning and if they did, I could go onto another hormone drug that would be more effective than Tamoxifen. If not, I'd have to stay on Tamoxifen, the most effective drug for menopausal women.

It was all strangely anti-climactic. I'm not sure how I expected to feel but driving home, I couldn't stop thinking: 'I don't have to do this anymore and I don't have to come back to this hospital until September.'

Liv kissed my forehead as we left, saying: 'Mummy, aren't you so pleased it's all over? No more hospital visits.'

When we got home, Iain cracked open the bottle of Ruinart which my mum asked him to buy for us, we had dinner and made a toast to good health.

It felt like karma that on this special day, as I was cleansing my face before bed, I noticed the first tiny eyebrow hairs poking through. It was like a reward for finishing. They looked like downy baby caterpillars sitting above my eyes. It was weird to see the first evidence of eyebrows on my face having got accustomed to seeing none at all. Along with the fluffy down covering my head, the journey back to normal had started. The blonde ones coming through on my chin I could have happily lived without. I looked like a new born chick, which felt quite apt.

And breathe… Swap coffee for pure organic green tea. It's an acquired taste but once you do it, you won't look back. It has anti-cancer properties and is being used in powerful new tumour treating drugs. Green tea with jasmine is delicious.

Chapter Twenty Three

An Email Entitled 'Drinking'

I've always believed that leading an active lifestyle, eating healthily and exercising regularly allowed me to eat and drink pretty much whatever I wanted in moderation so giving up wholemeal bread, the little dairy I ate, alcohol, chicken - the only meat I ate - and the odd cake was really hard. Going out for supper was tough unless I went off plan and I wasn't the only one struggling.

I met Abi through a mutual friend shortly after she had been diagnosed with malignant melanoma, a couple of months after my diagnosis. A young, sassy beautiful woman who kept fit, did Pilates and looked after herself, Abi was another example of cancer's unjust system of victim selection. She had also consulted Simone on an anti-cancer diet to do whatever she could to keep herself healthy and well following her operation. We were alike in many ways, even sharing the same birthday, and another thing we shared was the love of a good night out, which was not reflected in the food plan.

I sat down at my PC one morning ready to start work and saw an email from Abi entitled 'Drinking'.

'Karen, I've got a couple of big nights coming up and the thought of two glasses of wine doesn't really fill me with excitement,' she confessed. 'I know that's awful but I'm wondering what damage I'll do if I have more?' I had to laugh when I saw the subject bar.

When I changed my diet six months earlier, like Abi, I was determined to do everything by the letter and for the first few months, that's exactly what I did. I found it so hard but was really proud of myself. Then the cravings started...I had never been on a diet before so I had no idea that when you cut things out, they are exactly what you crave. No wonder weight loss plans fail all the time! Despite this, I lost seven kilos in weight and looked dreadful. I spoke to two close friends who had been on Simone's food plan – one was a sufferer of severe colitis and the other just wanted to lead a more healthy life. They both said they fell off the wagon and couldn't do the diet religiously but if I could stick to it five days a week, that was as much as I could hope for. I wanted to do everything 100% all the time but I realised this was never going to work and would eventually make me a grumpy, skinny, miserable bitch.

Of course, there were also weekends where I drank six weeks' worth of champagne in 48 hours but as long as you didn't hit the bottle every night, what harm would it do? So I told Abi to go for it, really enjoy herself on those special occasions and just drink plenty of water and keep taking the milk thistle tabs. Even when I cheated, my readings on Simone's tests were tip top considering the treatments I was enduring, probably because of all the supplements I was taking.

One advantage to cutting out sugar and alcohol was how much better my skin looked. Avoiding refined sugar makes a big difference to the elasticity and firmness of skin. Over the years I've spent fortunes on creams and serums but using Absolution, Natural Elements and Lierac oil and day cream could not be the only reason it was glowing and clear and best of all, fairly line free, after months of deathly pallor.

I had made permanent changes that I was determined to stick to...drinking water with lemon and cayenne first thing in the morning to neutralise toxins in my system, drinking more water in general and staying away from dairy and refined sugar for the most part. But on the occasional days when I fancied an almond croissant sprinkled copiously with icing sugar and a latte, I would have it and I finally stopped beating myself up about it. The journey was hard enough without all of life's little pleasures being snatched away.

I was reminded of that when I read another of Abi's emails recalling the up and down days after her surgery. 'I will never forget the nights I used to sneak into the kid's rooms and lie and hug them whilst sleeping and just cry,' she confided. 'And I couldn't really get angry with them for a long while - in fact I still find it hard now. And I remember my first post op hair wash and hair dry - it took me forever but there was such a great sense of achievement!'

I was so glad to be free of hospital constraints but I contacted Clooney after reading a ground-breaking new study in The Lancet which reported that a dose of 75mg a day of enteric coated aspirin had been proven in clinical trials to prevent as well as treat cancer. Not only does it stop cancers from growing in the first place, by preventing cancer cells from bonding to platelets, it also stops cancer from travelling around the body.

For five people taking aspirin, two have metastasis - the spread of cancer from one part of the body to another - prevented, according to the study. A small daily dose also cuts the risk of metastasis in patients who have only just started taking it. Aspirin was already known to reduce the risk of heart attacks and strokes and now it could help to beat cancer too.

It could also cause internal bleeding but I was happy to take my chances if it meant less of a risk of being stricken by cancer in the future. I emailed Clooney to ask what he thought and he emailed back immediately.

'No problem to take aspirin for your cancer,' he said. 'There are also benefits for the prevention of vascular disease.' I stopped by the pharmacy on the way home to stock up.

I was entering my non-treatment phase and it felt good. Sitting at my PC as the clock hit 4pm immersed in research, it was so refreshing not to have to drop everything, leg it to the car and drive to hospital. I sent an email to my friends to tell them that treatment had ended and amongst the lovely messages back was a fantastic video from my journalist friend Sarah M of her two boys, who had to be prised apart while scrapping over a bow and arrow to record a message for me. I cried for the first time in ages watching them chant: 'We're glad you're feeling better Karen.' But my tears soon turned to laughter when Sarah ordered them to smile at the end and these big forced grins appeared!

'It only took five takes, Kazza, and I was crying too – tears of rage,' she told me through gritted teeth.

For the first time in many months, I felt like celebrating so I invited a few friends over for lunch the day before leaving for Toronto to do the job that had kept me going through the dark days. There was no time to pack as I sweated in the kitchen making salmon and ginger fishcakes and a variety of salads and uncorked the first bottle of bubbly.

The sun shone, the pool, which was finally finished after five arduous and stressful months of work, was looking amazing (despite having sprung a small and irritating leak) and the Champagne flowed along with lovely words from all my friends. I toyed with the idea of going bareheaded but decided against it. Not because I didn't feel comfortable but because many people, even close friends, didn't know quite how to react to me.

There was a woman receiving treatment at my radiotherapy unit who always came in bald with no wig or hat on. I would stare at her out of admiration for the way she did her thing without worrying about attracting attention and wished I had her courage. I knew I would have to get used to going bare by the time we reached Venice Beach in Los Angeles at the end of the month as surfing in a wig was a no no.

I was more excited about this flight than any other and hastily threw together some warm and cold weather gear for the three week trip. I was starting in Toronto then spending a few days in London before heading off to the Coachella music festival in Palm Springs and surfing in LA.

I detest packing and it was a bigger pain than usual due to my fingernails having finally turned black underneath and feeling loose, painful and like they might fall off at any moment. Carrying out the most mundane tasks like opening and shutting a suitcase were suddenly very tricky. Having been housebound for so long, I was also a little nervous and lacking in confidence but none of this could take away the overwhelming joy at being a free agent once again.

It was emotional saying goodbye to the girls before Iain drove me to the airport. The girls grew up with me travelling abroad regularly on jobs so they were used to me jetting off but this time, they hugged me a little bit harder and longer, knowing what a milestone it was for me to reach this point. Iain was more direct. 'Just be careful please, especially with the surfing. Don't overdo it. Most of all, enjoy yourself,' he said as he hugged me close.

And breathe… Plan a reward for when your treatment ends. My trip was the light at the end of the tunnel that kept me going when I was at my lowest point.

Chapter Twenty Four

Back In The Saddle Again

The things that inspire us can be quite random. For me, it was seeing a teenage girl in pyjamas and a leg cast in a hospital waiting room, bald but still beautiful and wearing a little light make up and some great false lashes. She was clearly in the middle of chemotherapy and could not have been much older than 16 or 17, but there she was, boldly hobbling through a packed London hospital with no concern as to what anyone thought. She looked amazing and she was my inspiration for eventually daring to go bareheaded.

Meeting my PR friend Jakki at Heathrow Airport for our trip to cover Britain and Ireland's Next Top Model in Toronto was emotional. We had spent the previous 10 years hopping around the world together on jobs, working hard and playing hard whenever we had an afternoon off in an exotic location. We hadn't seen each other for several months and in line with my desire to keep my illness a secret from work colleagues, I had only just told her about my treatment. The last time I'd seen her, I had long blonde hair, so rocking up with a synthetic crop was never going to pass unnoticed. It felt right to fill her in. We hugged and she admired the wig.

The seven hour British Airways flight went smoothly as I sipped a glass of Champagne and watched the real George Clooney in The Descendants, a poignant tale of a woman whose fractured family comes to terms with their future as she lies in a coma in hospital following an accident. I would not advise watching it if even slightly depressed. Other passengers may have thought I had a bladder problem as I was getting up every 40 minutes or so to go to the loo so that I could take off my wig and scratch my poor itchy head and let it get some air before plopping the wig on again and wandering back to my seat.

We arrived at the Windsor Arms Hotel, reputed to be Madonna and the real Clooney's favourite hotel in the city, and it was easy to see why. Discreet friendly service in a historic townhouse in the heart of Yorkville, it boasted a rooftop gym and a butler's pantry straight from the room to the kitchen. You called room service and they left your order in it and switched on a light to let you know it was there. Very dangerous indeed.

My morning dilemma was not whether to do the pool and gym before breakfast but how. I couldn't swim in a wig and did not yet have enough hair to go bare, so I got into the habit of getting there at 7am. I suppose I could have chanced it but it was whether to swim bare and be paranoid every time I heard a noise, or swim with my swim cap on, which I hated but felt protected in. I chose the latter. Just as well because on the first morning, one of the other journalists on the trip appeared without warning, unable to sleep due to jet lag, and called out breezily: 'Morning Karen. What a great idea to bring a swimming cap – I really hate getting my hair wet too!'

I managed to stifle my laughter and carried on with 50 lengths followed by my first cycle ride in six months in the gym, conscious of the fact that the Piste to Plage Challenge was less than five months away. I'd been out of chemo for two months already and it was exactly a week since my last radiotherapy. I managed to cycle 10 miles and felt very pleased with myself.

Feeling refreshed, I met the other journalists for breakfast before heading off to explore Toronto ahead of meeting up with the show's presenter Elle Macpherson and the rest of the production team. It was a day of wig references, largely thanks to the journalist

I had bumped into that morning at the pool (who shall remain nameless to spare her blushes!)

The Canadian wind was blowing a hooley so I literally had to hold onto my hair for fear of it taking off across the block. Inexplicably, the conversation turned to who wears wigs in the showbiz world. My writer colleague named a few household names including Barbara Windsor, and when I expressed surprise, she said: 'It's very easy to tell. If there's no visible parting, it's always a wig!' The irony of me clinging onto my wig as she told me this was not lost on me.

Then she identified another wig giveaway - a hairless nape - before ruffling the back of my wig to demonstrate! How do people know these things? She seemed remarkably up the subject and I was laughing inside about how awful it would be if her fingers got stuck in the netting of my wig. I got away with it although I'm not sure how.

Later that afternoon, we headed to a chic city hotel in readiness for the interviews with Elle. I dash to the loo to try and rescue the windswept wig, which by now looked like it had just been dragged through Hurricane Katrina. I spent 15 minutes combing it through with my fingers in front of the mirror and making sure it wasn't crooked and didn't expose any bald bits. I also drew on my non-existent eyebrows with a soft brown Mac eye liner pencil. Every little bit helps.

Back at the lobby, I was ushered into the area where Elle and her assistant Donna were waiting. It's fair to say any normal woman would feel inadequate beside Elle. After all, we are talking about one of the world's most beautiful and successful supermodels. With her mane of long honey blonde hair, flawless skin and a toned body which belies her years, she looked absolutely drop dead gorgeous. I, on the other hand, did not. I felt physically sick with nerves. I found myself praying that my wig wouldn't move or end up crooked and my eyebrows wouldn't smudge or rub off completely. My skin was like dry parchment, wrinkled and paper thin, and I looked and felt every second of my 45 years.

Some of the production crew was also around. This was a location trip I had done every year for the last seven or eight years with the same team but clearly losing weight and wearing a wig in place of my usual long blonde locks had transformed me, and not in a good way. Elle, her assistant and the rest of the production team didn't recognise me at first. When it dawned on them that it was me, there was a barrage of, 'Nice haircut, really suits you,' type comments, which was sweet but made me wish for the day when I could go out skinhead length all over and look like a butch lesbian instead of wearing a bloody blonde ferret.

Chatting to Elle was a sobering experience. She makes mere mortals like me feel like a fully loaded dumper truck with or without hair. It felt quite surreal to be sitting there feeling so old, pinched and unattractive next to one of the world's most beautiful women. There were quite a few times during my illness when I would have happily put the clock forward six months in order to be looking vaguely normal and like me again. This was one of them. I decided not to mention my illness. It felt irrelevant as well as not very professional to steal the thunder from your subject. Within minutes, Elle and I were chatting away and I forgot my concerns. It ended up being a great interview and made me feel like I was back in the game again.

A couple of nights into the trip, the press gang were out for supper at a cosy little Italian and the subject of hair came up again. I mentioned that my usual style was a lot longer and my hair-obsessed colleague fixed me with a look and said: 'Yes, I've been thinking about your hair a lot. You never seem to have one strand out of place. How do you do it?'

This time, I couldn't continue the deception and quietly told her the truth. Poor thing, she was hugely embarrassed and concerned but I couldn't help seeing the funny side of us spending three days talking about very little else apart from my hair. It was a big thing to share with someone I didn't know very well but I was starting to relax about people knowing the truth of what I'd been through. The following morning I felt comfortable enough to swim without my cap and kept it off in the sauna as there was no one else there. It was liberating.

Returning home to the UK for a few days before heading to Los Angeles, I had the chance to catch up with friends and family. As I tucked into an Indian takeaway one evening with some girlfriends, Susie took me aside, gave me a bear hug and said: 'You look like the old you again. When I hugged you last Christmas, you were so thin I thought you might break.'

I showed them my sprouting hair, which was coming through darker than I'd ever seen it, and Susie added: 'Just lose the wig, you look great with no hair.'

When to go wigless had become my new dilemma. My hair was very fine and downy with odd longer hairs dotted about and yet strangely I looked more like me without a wig than with it.

My mum had to go for X-rays and a consultation at a London hospital so I went with her. I noticed a stark contrast between the NHS and the French healthcare system. Each waiting room was packed with patients, so much so that there was an overspill of people standing in corridors waiting. The X-rays took almost an hour and the follow up consultation happened 90 minutes after mum's allotted appointment time.

As I glanced around at other patients trying to pass the time, I spotted the teenage cancer patient on crutches in a leg cast, making her way to the reception desk accompanied by her mum. Her head was completely shiny and hair-free as a result of ongoing chemotherapy. I couldn't help but marvel at her bravery to go bare, with not a care for what anyone else thought, and instantly made a decision to do the same.

Arriving at a friend's house in North London for drinks, I decided it was time to dispense with the wig forever. I took it off as soon as I walked through the front door and felt an overwhelming sense of liberation. I was quite comfortable without it but often forgot that the sight of me bald was a shock for other people.

Heading out for supper, I was fortified by the sight of the brave teenager I saw in hospital. It was impossible to plan for a moment like this, it had to be spontaneous, which was why my proposed bald shopping trip to Cannes fell apart. I wanted to do it but when it came to it, I lost my bottle. Suddenly, I felt brave. It was time to stop worrying about what other people thought and quit shielding everyone from the reality of what had happened to me.

Strolling up the road in the fresh night air and feeling the chill on my head felt good. Walking into the restaurant, I noticed the manager and the waiter immediately avert their eyes. They found it hard to look at me. Seeing a bald, middle-aged woman is clearly a taboo and looking directly at one is not the done thing. It gave me a very small idea of what it must be like to be disabled. People are so afraid of staring at you or offending you that they would rather play safe by not engaging at all and simply ignore you, addressing everyone else but you.

We sat down and ordered some drinks and rather meanly, I made strenuous efforts to catch the waiter's eye. By the time we ordered mint tea after supper, he was finally able to look me in the eye for the first time. I didn't feel awkward. I was far more embarrassed wearing the wig, as it had always felt crooked and weird, like a family of river creatures nesting on my head. I felt liberated as we left the restaurant in gale force winds and rain.

The wig was packed into the bottom of my suitcase and the next day I set off for Heathrow Airport for my trip to Los Angeles with my girlfriends. I thought about throwing it away in a grand gesture of defiance but a little voice in my head said: 'Don't jinx it.'

Walking from the car to Paddington station in the rain, I noticed that no one really looked at me. Not standing out was a good feeling. Walking through Terminal 3 to meet the girls was a breeze, and when I stopped by the Dr Sebagh counter at Duty Free to reapply some eye cream (as my eyes were weeping a lot through a lack of lashes) the beauty girls heaped free samples on me, even though I didn't buy anything. Result!

Arriving in LA after the 11 hour Virgin flight, the passport queue was about 200 people deep, which would have meant at least an hour's wait, but the nice security lady took one look at me and whisked us to the front. The cancer card was finally coming good.

And breathe….There is a lot of crappy stuff that comes with cancer but one of the best discoveries was the kindness of strangers.

Chapter Twenty Five

Surfing USA

One of the things that became very important to me when I first became ill was having something to look forward to whenever it all felt like it was getting too much. Planning jobs and holidays had a therapeutic and positive effect, keeping me sane at times when I felt like screaming with frustration. After months of anticipation and will-they-won't-they let me go, it felt good to have made it to Los Angeles.

Throughout my treatment, the prospect of my LA trip kept me going. Whenever I was in pain or feeling a little bit down, I thought about surfing in the crashing waves, shopping and brunching in West Hollywood and having a laugh with my friends. We had a few minor problems strapping Sarah's surfboard to the roof of our hired Jeep on arrival, so the girls had to hang onto the roof straps all the way to our hotel in West Hollywood. The great thing about having a surfboard strapped to the roof is that you can always identify your hire car in a busy multi-storey car park. And it was even easier to spot once we arrived in Palm Springs. I mean who brings a surfboard to the desert?

Armed with my floppy sun hat, high factor sun screen and my happy face, we made our way to the Coachella Festival, and by 11am it was already touching 110 degrees, which meant keeping a hat on my bald head at all times. The highlights were the Arctic Monkeys, Black Keys, Madness, Pulp and Swedish House Mafia and that was just day one. But a scare the following day served as a warning not to try and be superwoman. We were in one of the tents watching Kasabian thrill the crowd and the atmosphere was electric. It was packed and the extraordinary heat meant there was very little air and a lot of dust.

Suddenly, I started getting into difficulty breathing. Every time I tried to take a breath, a sharp pain stabbed my right side, just under my breast bone. I stayed in the tent as I didn't want to lose my friends amongst the huge crowd but as soon as the band finished playing, the girls helped me stagger outside for some air. The pain refused to subside and after an hour of sitting quietly on the grass surrounded by worried faces, we decided to call it a night.

I thought a good night's sleep might cure me but I woke up the next morning still struggling to breathe and the pain had moved round to my right shoulder blade. After all my treatment, the idea of spending a precious day of my holidays seeing doctors and having scans did not appeal. I was angry about falling ill again following so much treatment. It felt so unfair. Painkillers helped and after a chat with my doctor friend in London, I decided to wait and see my GP once I was back home. It looked for a while like the idea of surfing, the light at the end of my tunnel, had been extinguished, but when the pain dissipated three days later just as we arrived on the coast, I decided to tentatively give it a go.

I rented a surf board and wetsuit across the road from our hotel in Venice and Sarah and I headed for the beach. The sea was freezing but running into the breakers and catching my first wave felt every bit as good as I had imagined it would during the dark days. I'd had lots of lectures from my friends and Iain about not overdoing it but daily swim sessions at our hotel helped to build my stamina to the point that after two hours and many great waves, I quit only through numb feet rather than fatigue. It was the first time I felt smug about having no hair: for once, I didn't miss any waves trying to see through sea matted strands plastered across my face.

I made sure I stayed warm and didn't outstay my welcome in the water and my breathing didn't deteriorate. It was the biggest buzz

I'd had since I got ill. Simone had told me that positive energy is cancer's enemy so I enjoyed another surf session the following day.

Maybe it was the warm sunshine but my hair had started growing like crazy. Three months after finishing chemo, I was sporting a proper hairline once more, a very thin, very dark covering of hair. I had already started Veeting my bikini line, which was growing faster than the hair on my head. The injustice!

The reaction I received in LA was overwhelmingly positive. One girl came up to me by the hotel pool to tell me I was a babe and a guy at the festival shouted out: 'Cool hair lady!' It was liberating to note that the wig had spent an entire week in my suitcase, squashed under shiny new purchases.

I was so used to my appearance by now that I forgot what a shock it was to friends who hadn't seen me in a while. One old film PR friend came to pick me up at Venice Beach so we could catch up. The last time I'd seen her we were living it up after Cannes Film Festival. She drew up to my hotel in her car and as I jumped in, she burst into tears.

'You look great,' she sobbed, hugging me hard. 'Just different.'

It was a pleasure to arrive back in France after three weeks away. Combining interviews, fun, surfing, regular workouts and great gigs was fun and a bit tiring but I was amazed at how well my body had withstood the onslaught given that it was less than four weeks since my treatment had ended. My girlfriends, or fellow Desert Dogs, as we became known, were more tired than I was.

Having got used to walking around bald in Los Angeles, it was a big test to come back and do the same on home turf. When you are thousands of miles from home and know nobody, it's far easier than arriving at your friends' houses or going to your local eatery looking like a boy, and a bald one at that.

Meeting an old friend and her new boyfriend for dinner was my first test. Iain was away and it was the first time I had been out on my own without the comfort and protection of my friends around me, and to a restaurant I regularly go to. I felt nervous so I dressed up, put on some eye liner and looked for my mascara. I hadn't been able to wear it for months and once I had located it hidden away in one of the girl's make up bags (they have no shame), I was ready to face the world. Well, Valbonne at least. If people stared as I walked across the busy square, which was packed with tourists and diners, it wasn't immediately obvious. My friend's boyfriend was charming and pretty soon, we were laughing and chatting and I had forgotten all about what a big deal it was to get myself out of the house.

My confidence was returning and I noticed that when friends and acquaintances saw me out and about, there was an initial look of surprise that I was daring to go wigless, and then pride that I was brave enough to face the world without hiding behind a wig.

The breathing pains were consistent but not debilitating so I drove to see my GP. We chatted and he told me how well I looked before listening to my breathing, testing my lung capacity and trying me out with some inhalers in case my childhood asthma had flared up again. Finally, he suggested a chest scan.

'Why don't you pop down to the hospital now for a chest X-ray?' he added, writing out the prescriptions for a scan and an X-ray.

'At least that will show up anything serious in advance of the scan.'

'What are you thinking it might be?' I asked nervously.

He peered at me over his spectacles. 'Well, a pulmonary embolism is possible.'

'Could it be anything to do with the cancer?' I asked, barely daring to breathe. This was my fear, that somehow despite the clear scans of a few months ago, something had developed or spread to the lung area.

'Very unlikely given that everything was clear when they discharged you,' he added, which meant I could breathe again.

I jumped in the car and drove to hospital. At the radiology department, I checked in with the admin clerk and handed over my prescription. Within five minutes, I was called into the radiography room and X-rayed. Less than 10 minutes later I had my results in my hand. I've never been so pleased to see the words 'normale' and 'libre'. It was not a pulmonary embolism, which was a huge relief.

The girls were off school and decided they would accompany me to hospital for my chest scan a couple of days later. To make it a bit more exciting for them, I took them clothes shopping and popped into the optician to get my sunglasses fixed. A few stares came my way but I barely noticed them. The salesman cheerfully fixed a new screw in my Ralph Lauren glasses and wouldn't charge me.

'Result mum, maybe he felt sorry for you,' said Issy. 'Do you think we'll get lunch for free too?

We stopped off at the hospital on the way back for my CT scan. It took an hour and half and I had to inhale radioactive gas through my mouth for a minute - deeply unpleasant - and lie under a scanner for 15 minutes, keeping perfectly still while the scanner rotated around my chest. Then the male nurse injected me with a radioactive substance and the scanner revolved again for another 15 minutes. Finally I was submerged in the tube while it spun around me. I felt like Jodie Foster in Contact. A sign on the scanner said: 'Do not look at the laser beam', so, of course, that is exactly what I wanted to do.

The wait to see the doctor for the results felt like forever. I tried to think positively but I was so used to getting bad news after scans that mentally I was all over the place, while trying to stay outwardly calm for the sake of the girls, who were keeping boredom at bay by playing on their iPads in the waiting room.

They changed the screensaver on my phone from a photo of the dogs to a picture of them smiling in their new furry Cossack hats on Christmas Day. Last Christmas was my worst ever but I spent the wait for my results looking at their happy little faces and hoping that this Christmas would be better.

Finally, the doctor explained my results...nothing suspicious, no sign of pulmonary embolism or pleurisy and the pains were probably as a result of the radiotherapy. I just had to be patient and wait for it to clear up by itself.

And breathe...Get used to every little health niggle signalling a return of the dreaded C word. It doesn't, of course, but just try convincing your irrational brain of that fact.

Chapter Twenty Six

Film Festival Glamour And Me

The Cannes Film Festival is the most glamorous event of the showbiz year by a country mile. The world's biggest designers clamour to dress Hollywood and European A-listers for the red carpet and everyone is coiffed and made up to the nines for the premieres, parties and after parties along the Croisette. It's fair to say the idea of mingling with Tinseltown's finest on superyachts and in stunning party locations looking like I'd just been scalped was not appealing. But work is work and after months of doing very little, I was prepared to take a deep breath and get on with it.

Following my breathing problems, my doctors had strongly advised me against too much exercise, which threw the Piste to Plage challenge into disarray. I reluctantly phoned the organisers to tell them that I could not take part in the four day bike ride through the French Alps in September. I'm not sure who was more gutted, me or them. I so hoped to do it but given the fact that in the space of four months I had to achieve near superhuman fitness from a below par starting point, it would have been total madness.

They came up with a very worthwhile compromise - driving up to the start point on Day Four in the alpine resort of Auron and completing the final ride, 111 km down to the coast at Juan-les-

Pins, with the rest of the riders. Given that the final day fell on the first anniversary of my cancer diagnosis, it was a good alternative and a way of marking an anniversary with a defiant punch in the air without putting my body under too much strain. Even so, once we finished the conversation, I hung up and went out for a run and shed a few tears at the disappointment of not being able to do the whole ride.

I came home, wiped away my tears and decided to set up a fund raising page, explaining why I was taking part in the challenge and what it meant to me. If ever I needed a boost, it was then, and it came in the shape of many wonderful messages and donations from friends and colleagues, many of whom were unaware of my illness.

It was also a relief to put the information out there finally and not have to have upsetting conversations with people I hadn't spoken to about what I'd been going through. It felt like a great weight had been lifted from my shoulders.

I started Tamoxifen, one tab a day to keep the doctor at bay, and had no side effects apart from the odd hot flush. There was only one screaming match at home, which didn't involve me, and no mood swings, depression or weight gain.

My look at this point could best be described as GI Jane. The soft downy thatch had grown to 5mm all over by mid-May and included quite a few greys but I was loathe to pull any of them out as I had so little. At least they were all firmly attached, I kept tugging at the ends to make sure. Having hair on my head rather than my pillow was a novelty, as was using a pea sized amount of shampoo and conditioner again after months of not needing to bother. The fact that it was growing back a rather disturbing shade of dark grey was a shock but I hadn't seen my true hair colour in 25 years so no wonder it looked unfamiliar.

The Cannes Film Festival was fast approaching and I felt quite daunted about the prospect of covering it. My index fingernail was the first to fall off, leaving a very deformed and discoloured new nail in its wake. The others were starting to lift too. I confided my glamour worries to my friend Susie, who said, 'Why don't you just wear your wig to the parties?' But that would have felt like taking a step backwards. Wearing the wig would still mean a bad hair day as

I hated it, far better to brave the quizzical looks and exploit the fact that no celeb in the world was going to refuse to talk to me looking like this. I decided I'd rather have my own bad hair than someone else's.

To take my mind off things, I went for a gentle 5 km run in warm sunshine. The heavy scent of orange blossom and jasmine hung in the valley like a veil and it was the most enriching, enlivening feeling, running through that heady fragrance towards the hills. Despite the trials of the previous eight months, I was feeling good. We were invited to the Historic Grand Prix in Monte-Carlo to watch a friend racing his classic car, which meant a ridiculously early start to catch a train to Monaco. Our efforts were rewarded when we reached the port at Monte-Carlo to be met by a motor launch which took us to a beautiful yacht moored right by the track. We enjoyed coffee and breakfast on board and spent the next few hours getting an ear bashing of the loveliest kind from all the amazing race cars zooming around the track.

When the clouds burst in a sudden downpour, I was the one laughing loudest as my hair didn't go frizzy or hang limply down my back in the storm, neither did it get blown into something resembling an unsprung mattress on the yacht. It simply looked slick and quite edgy. It was a win-win and a successful practice run for Cannes.

On the first day of Film Festival, I headed into town to watch the press screening of the opening film Moonrise Kingdom. The mood on the red carpet was buoyant with Bruce Willis, Tilda Swinton, Ed Norton, Bill Murray and Jason Schwartzman joshing around and playing up to the hundreds of cameras pointing in their direction.

Afterwards, I headed off to Nikki Beach Club to meet a PR contact and bumped into a lovely (bald) editor from GQ in New York. We chatted and he told me that no one ever forgets him because he is bald. It's fair to say that he and I looked very different to the rest of the clientele at the bar, who were mainly bleached and natural blondes with long tresses swinging down their backs. If I'm honest, I succumbed to a little bit of follicle envy. It was hard being the boyish one surrounded by dozens of perfectly groomed beautiful women wherever I looked. Hell, even the men had more hair than I did!

The film parties were in full swing and I was going with the flow, attending as many as I could fit in to report back for the UK and US magazines I was working for. It's a pinch-me-I'm-dreaming moment when you are on a superyacht surrounded by the likes of Alec Baldwin and Eva Longoria, blow-dried to within an inch of their lives, sipping Champagne as the DJ spins tunes on the deck and a groaning table of delicious tiny canapés beckons.

To hell with the food plan tonight, I thought, as I dived into a whipped seafood mousse and sipped a glass of Veuve Cliquot. This was as glamorous as Film Festival gets but before you scream with envy, I will let you into a little secret. The truth was that it was freezing, the party girls in barely there cocktail dresses were shivering and there was lots of polite small talk going on amongst the assembled exclusive clique of celebs, film production people, professional party people and hangers on. Lots of middle aged film financiers were also trying to dance.

My job that night was to watch and see who turned up and try not to freeze to death in the process. My feet were so cold that at least my heels didn't hurt when I put them back on again. The rule of thumb is everyone removes their shoes before going on board, even Eva Longoria, who was even more tiny than usual without hers.

I bumped into a number of work colleagues during the course of the festival. There was always a look of surprise when they finally realised it was me. Hair defines a person, giving you something to hide behind, play with and be identified by. Some people were direct in asking what was wrong, others were less forthcoming.

I was proud of the fact that I was strong enough to brave the glamour and go bare. Even rapper Jay-Z, who I bumped into at Kanye West's film premiere party, complimented my style. All eyes were on Kanye and Kim Kardashian, who were lovingly swaying together in time to the music in a VIP area just by the pool at the Palm Beach so I couldn't believe my eyes when I spotted Jay-Z all alone, shimmying on the spot to the disco classic All Night Long right next to me, with his minders a respectable distance away.

'It's Jay-Z isn't it?' I said and he held out his hand and said, 'Yes maam,' shaking mine. We started chatting about how long he was in town for and how much he and Beyoncé love Cannes then, out of the blue, he piped up with: 'I am loving your hair.' This wasn't the time to tell him it wasn't out of choice so I graciously accepted the compliment with, 'Thanks, it's very easy, I just wash and go.'

'Hey, tell me about it!' he grinned, rubbing his own close crop and we both laughed. Jay-Z was the only celebrity during the Film Festival who had the chutzpah to comment on my hair. No-one else went there.

As the days rolled by, my confidence in my appearance increased and interviews with Dr Who actress Karen Gillan, who recently shaved her head for a film role, Keith Lemon and Kelly Brook went swimmingly, although I often wondered what they were really thinking when they saw a middle-aged female skinhead rock up to interview them. Whatever they thought, they kept it to themselves.

I survived the Cannes Film Festival running between interviews, screenings and parties for 12 days and wasn't sure just how I would pull it off as no bedtime came before 3.30am. I felt great, if a bit jaded. Highlight number one was watching Brad Pitt, who looked gorgeous on the red carpet at the premiere for his gangster movie Killing Them Softly, and a close second was drinking two months rations of bubbly at the parties. Calvin Klein's party was the ritziest, at a sumptuous villa above Super Cannes with Ben Stiller, Naomi Watts, Jessica Chastain, Hayley Atwell and Lara Stone amongst the guests. I had a long chat with Hayley over a glass of Moet. We talked about the craziness of Cannes, her upcoming film roles and the glorious over-the-top-ness of the parties.

The Filmmaker's dinner at the exclusive Hotel du Cap Eden Roc was also a glamorous affair. Robert de Niro was there with his wife Grace Hightower along with Ray Liotta, Karolina Kurkova, Skyfall actress Berenice Marlohe, Terry Gilliam, Eric Dane and Gerard Butler. I chatted to Ewan McGregor, who brought his mum Carole along with his wife Eve. Again, no mention of my less than flattering steely skinhead.

Ronnie Wood was electric at a private gig at the VIP Room on the

Croisette but by day nine I was starting to flag. Iain suggested a pizza with the girls just outside our village and I jumped at the chance to eat something more substantial than the delicate lobster and prawn canapés and sushi that are de rigueur at all the parties. We were in the car on the way to the pizzeria when my mobile rang. It was a PR asking if I would like to attend a gala dinner that night at the Carlton Hotel for The Paperboy movie, where I would be sitting alongside Nicole Kidman, John Cusack, Matthew McConaughey and Zac Efron. I looked down at my jeans, Converse and T shirt and let them know that actually, I had other plans. It occurred to me that three months earlier, I wouldn't have lasted one night on the town, let alone nine. It was time to let the stars party without me.

I planned to get back on the wagon as soon as possible, cutting out alcohol, drinking lots of water and getting plenty of sleep. In the spirit of doing things right, when I felt peckish midway through writing up an interview, I baked a batch of cereal bars rather than raid the biscuit tin. I was tucking into one when I crunched on something a lot harder than a macadamia nut. It was half my tooth, which had broken clean away from a molar at the top of my mouth. I rang my dentist and told her about my problem and my treatment and she kindly fitted me in for an emergency appointment.

Chemotherapy upsets the balance of bacteria in the mouth and I was told there was no doubt that this previously healthy tooth was weakened by all the drugs in my system. Coming out of treatment was so exciting that I forgot that the after-effects can continue for months on end. Four appointments and €800 later, it looked perfect again and I made a mental note to lay off the nuts when I baked the next batch of cereal bars.

And breathe…I think Kate Moss missed the point when she said, 'Nothing tastes as good as skinny feels.' I have my own take on that. Nothing feels as good as normal feels. You don't miss normal until it's gone.

Chapter Twenty Seven

Summer Breeze

The sun was shining and I felt the best I'd felt in many months. I was trying to listen to the voice in my head telling me to take it slow. It was tough as I was so much stronger and had more energy than I'd had in months but I noticed that on the days when I listened to that little voice and left my phone and computer alone and didn't overdo it, I reaped the benefits.

Normal life, the thing I had hankered after for so long, resumed at breakneck pace. I swam at the beach, lunched and dined with friends, drank wine and made merry into the early hours and embarked on as much work as I could generate with gusto.

There was a little voice in my head, however, that was urging caution and warning me not to overdo it and I tried to listen. I could see how easy it would be PC to fall headlong back into bad old habits and revert back to the life I lived BC. Not that there was a lot wrong with that life but I promised myself that I would carry through at least some of the changes I had made during treatment. Chiefly, not drinking so much alcohol, saying no more often, keeping stress at bay and sticking to the basic food principles that had kept me so well during chemotherapy and had enabled my recuperation to be much speedier than expected. But with friends arriving every week and dinner and beach plans being made, it was proving harder than I thought, and it was all too easy to go with the flow.

On the morning of an important work deadline, I was tested to the limit. I had just settled down with a cup of green tea to email across copy to several magazines when my wireless switch inexplicably stopped working on my computer, leaving me with no internet connection. I could feel the panic rising at the anxiety of racing against the clock to get the problem sorted but I forced myself to calm down because panicking would not make it happen. Iain spent an hour fiddling with the settings before finding me a cable to plug directly into the internet box. It added an hour of precious time to my deadlines but they were completed and I managed not to lose my cool. As a reward, I left my phone and watch in the house and sat by the pool for almost two hours with a magazine. Not being able to check the time or emails was a gift.

I was rushing around the supermarket a few days later when I sped past a young mum with a toddler in her shopping trolley. The little girl stared at me before saying loudly: 'C'est pas une dame, Maman,' much to the mum's acute embarrassment. I could hear her shushing her daughter as I scooted into the next aisle and it dawned on me that although I had more hair than I'd had for seven months - think fluffy Mia Farrow - I really should remember to put on a little make up and jewellery when leaving the house if I didn't want to be mistaken for a bloke.

Following a fleeting 24 hour trip to London with delays both sides for work, I was feeling more tired than usual. A friend noticed and warned me to slow down. I had been planning my diary for the Monte-Carlo TV Festival and was accepting numerous invitations to parties, lunches and launches but with my friend's words ringing in my ears, I turned down a fabulous showbiz lunch so that I didn't have to make a three hour round trip. It was hard to type, 'Sorry I can't make it, I have a deadline,' but it was true insomuch as the deadline was my mental and physical health. So I listened to the little voice, did what I could and rested when I felt tired. Simple, and it worked.

When my Fleet Street friends came to visit several months earlier, I was a month into my chemotherapy, my hair was falling out and

I had lost several kilos in weight. In short, I didn't look great and staying firmly rooted in denial of how rubbish I was feeling was my modus operandi.

With a birthday party in Suffolk bringing us all together again for the first time since then, I was determined to look my best. I put some product into my fluffy short dark crop to make it look less post chemo and more intentional, spent far longer than usual on my make-up and donned a chic little black silk dress and my highest Prada wedges. When Sarah M walked into the room and gave me a polite smile, before doing a double take and racing across the room to give me a bear hug, I knew the effort had been worth it.

'Oh my God, I didn't recognise you, your hair looks AMAZING...you look AMAZING!' she squealed. 'You look so much better than the last time I saw you, even though you didn't actually ever look that bad.'

Other guests came up to me during the course of the evening to say they loved my hair. When you are feeling a bit self-conscious and plain compared to all the long haired glamour pusses around you, there's nothing like a compliment from a stranger to lift your sense of self-worth sky high.

We spent the weekend dancing in the field outside the house, drinking Champagne and catching up over endless cups of green tea and it was the best tonic anyone could possibly prescribe. For anyone who has been seriously ill, I advise a weekend in the bosom of your closest friends, drinking and laughing. It's as good, if not better, than any medicine. I chatted to one guest who had battled breast cancer four years ago. She put herself on a strict dairy free diet and looked amazing.

'When I saw you, I thought, there's someone else who has been through the mill,' she told me the following morning over breakfast. 'But you look great so I could see you were coming out the other side.'

She told me that one of the best things to come out of her illness was the fact that she didn't worry any more. 'I feel much more mellow and relaxed and silly little things do not get to me the way they used to,' she admitted.

Her husband, a former government medical officer, told me he believed the four best cancer fighting, tumour shrinking foods are turmeric, broccoli, green tea and pomegranate.

Rosé wasn't mentioned in his list, which was a shame as I drank lots of this while making lists about lists so that we forgot nothing when we left for a six week summer road trip around Europe. And when Iain and his brother Gary, who was staying with us, came back from two hours at the bar one evening, I just didn't want to miss out and joined them in a few glasses. Then I remembered that I had to see my GP before we left for some check-ups and guiltily glugged a couple of litres of water to dilute the Minuty rosé swilling around my bloodstream.

I had a good incentive for climbing back on the wagon as I was planning to start my cycling training in earnest as soon as we arrived at our first stop-off in Spain. My debut training ride was 24 km. It felt brilliant and even though my bottom ached, I was filled with a great sense of achievement despite the fact that it took me six minutes at a time to click my cycling shoes into the cleats on the pedals. I was not going to be a threat to anyone, in fact my main concern was whether I would be able to keep up on race day knowing that some of the other Piste to Plage riders were already knocking off 100 km on a typical training ride.

My second ride went well up to a point. That is, the point at which I fell off. Cycling 30 km in 30 degrees at 9am down the coastal road to the neighbouring village of Santa Pola was lovely, with the warm sea breeze stopping me from overheating. Confidence is not always a good thing though and when I decided to do a U-turn, I came unstuck, the dirt path loomed up ahead of me and unable to click my cleats out of the pedals in time, I collapsed in a heap as the bike landed on top of me. My first thought was did anyone see me? Luckily not. Only my pride was dented and my injuries - a rather lovely purple bruise on my left thigh and a deep scrape under my elbow - were superficial.

Whizzing along past little coves and beach bars was a wonderful way to explore the local area near our base on the east coast. There were plenty of hills but in the spirit of being on holiday, who needs a steep gradient when you can choose a gently sloping beachside plateau instead? It was perfect for a beginner like me, with gentle sweeping bends, fairly flat roads and beautiful scenery.

Taking off my cycling helmet, my hair - all mussed, sweaty and unstyled - sat in mad clumps giving me the appearance of a person who had just been released from a secure unit. Gary charged up his hair clippers and whizzed off the fluffy bits at the back of my neck and the straggly unattractive bits on my sideburns, making me look just a little more chic.

In addition to cycling, I got into the habit of heading off to the beach in the late afternoon, once the intense heat had died down, and going for a long swim in the sea. On the days when the wind was up and we had waves, we headed off with boogie boards and spent hours in the surf body boarding. It was the best feeling in the world, I could feel my lung capacity and energy levels improving every time. Taking life slowly, relaxing, doing as much exercise as I felt comfortable with and enjoying the holiday vibe was doing me the power of good.

Swimming, showering and hanging out in hot temperatures was much more pleasant thanks to the lack of hair. The vast majority of my friends and family told me to keep my hair short saying, 'You are so lucky it suits you,' but the girls wanted me to grow it back to how it was BC and part of me also wanted to look like I looked before. Flicking through a magazine on the beach, I saw a photograph of Anne Hathaway sporting a dark crop not dissimilar to mine. Well, with a few less grey hairs than me but she looked very chic and gave me confidence that cool women were opting for short urchin crops not unlike mine.

And breathe... I know I've said this already but it's so important it needs to be said again. Eat more pomegranates and broccoli and add turmeric to soups, casseroles and curries....along with green tea, these four are major anti-carcinogenic cancer fighting ingredients.

Chapter Twenty Eight

Chemo Brain Drain

One in four cancer survivors suffer from chemo brain - lack of memory, terrible concentration and increased clumsiness - after treatment. This was me (I think I've told you this before.) Trouble seemed to come and find me and by the end of our summer holiday, I was covered in cuts, bruises and stitches that this time had nothing to do with surgery. I discovered there's a lot to be said for taking your time, trusting your instincts and not hanging around for one last wave.

There is a reason I'm married to Iain, apart from the fact that he is the love of my life. I drive the car into posts, he rolls his eyes and patiently fixes it. I pack virtually everything I own (one case just for shoes, another for toiletries, you get my drift) while he travels light. I love a lie in while he is up before morning birdsong and has walked the dogs, had a coffee and prepared breakfast before I have even rubbed the sleep from my eyes.

We left Spain after two restful weeks for Arcachon and Cap Ferret in western France and our last evening before departing was spent in a frenzy of packing as Issy and I, who had oversized suitcases (so much her mother's daughter) waded through unworn, still folded clothes that there was no point in unpacking, or indeed packing in the first place, while Iain nonchalantly chucked a few bits into his diddy Samsonite and hey presto, he was off to the bar. Our plan for summer was a relaxing holiday with some work and adventure thrown in, but as usual, it was more eventful than we anticipated. I fell off my bike for the second time in front of 200 tourists as I left the ferry at Cap Ferret. It was far worse than landing in the dirt in Spain when at least no one else was around. A kind French guy hurried over to help me as I lay there thinking, if I can't cycle along a flat wooden jetty, what hope is there for me on steep mountain passes?

But the worst accident I had was while surfing at Biscarrosse near Bordeaux. I was catching some great waves and enjoying the water. After a couple of hours, I decided to get 'one last wave.' Famous last words. Unfortunately so did the guy next to me and he ploughed into me on his board, knocking me off my board and somehow entangling his ankle leash around my neck under the water. As I fought to release the cord and get out from underneath the board, the guy was tugging his board above me and strangling me. The surfboard fin smashed into the back of my ear and I finally emerged from the waves struggling for breath and choking on sea water, covered in blood, my diamond earring ripped from my earlobe and the back of my ear hanging open in a gaping slice.

The Baywatch guys spotted me staggering unsteadily out of the water as the debutante surfer followed behind me muttering abject apologies in French. They swung into action, speeding across the beach in their four wheel drive and hauling me into the front seat. Other bathers looked on in horror as my ear poured with blood all over the footwell in the car.

'You 'ave to 'ave stitches,' said David Hasselhoff as he led me into the first aid hut at the top of the beach and bathed my ear in antiseptic as I tried not to cry. I was sent off to Dr Fabian, a cool hippie with a surfboard in the corner of his surgery in town who apparently does a roaring trade stitching up all the middle aged surfing wannabes. The surf shop owner told me: 'Fabian is good with a needle and thread,' which was a relief to hear.

Fab Dr Fab took a photo of my wound with his iPhone to show me before and after, and following six neat stitches, he sighed: 'It's a shame it's behind the ear as it looks so pretty now. I am very proud of my work.' I was banned from the water until it healed.

When my poor mum heard what had happened, she urged me to take up a less hazardous sport than cycling or surfing, her suggestion being knitting.

Her words were still ringing in my ears when, on the UK leg of our road trip, we had a car crash on the motorway. The driver in front of us stopped dead in the fast lane for no apparent reason, and while we managed to pull up just in the nick of time, the van behind us didn't and ploughed straight into the back of our Jeep and my Canyon bike, which was strapped to the boot.

'There goes your bike,' said Iain as we jolted forwards with the impact of the crash. We drove over to the hard shoulder and despite the fact that it was a miracle no-one was hurt and more cars weren't involved, I found myself whimpering to the burly van driver as I looked at the tangled mess of metal hanging off the bike rack.

'I'm riding in a race in less than a month,' I cried, unable to stop my tears at the sheer unfairness of my cycling training being stopped by yet another pesky problem.

'Sorry love, nothing I could do,' he shrugged. 'What was that other guy playing at stopping dead like that?'

It felt like someone was trying to tell me something. Iain wanted to strap me into a straitjacket and put me in a dark room. But every time some crazy accident or injury struck, it only served to make me even more determined to keep going.

Flicking through the pages of Vogue on a non-active, non-biking, non-crashing day, I saw that it was all about the peroxide blonde crop, which was just as well as this precise look was my first proper post chemo hairstyle. When I lost my hair, I dreamed of the day I would have enough to have a short funky crop that didn't fall onto my shoulders every time I moved. The fact that it went orange first merely added to the drama. My hairdresser friend Karin looked even more alarmed than I did.

'Well, we were going for ash blonde….' she said pensively as she washed off the tint to reveal hair the colour of Rupert Grint's in Harry Potter. 'Don't worry, it's nothing a few highlights can't sort out,' she added quickly. An emergency rescue mission was mounted and 24 hours later, thanks to her expertise and calmness under pressure, I was sporting the edgy blonde crop I dreamed of all those months ago. Think Miley Cyrus crossed with Annie Lennox and you are close.

Three days later, I got the proof that I finally looked normal again. I was walking through the West End on the way to meet some work friends for supper when a guy came running up behind me.

'Excuse me, can I talk to you?' he puffed. 'I'm a photographer and I'm wondering if you'd like to do some modelling shots?'

'Are you having a laugh?' I said in disbelief, looking around for a hidden camera. 'I'm 45, and 5ft 4 inches tall. I'm not exactly Kate Moss.'

'What's that got to do with it?' he shot back, rustling in his wallet to hand me a business card. 'I think you have a really strong, unusual look, you are very confident and I love your bleached blonde crop. Please have a think and give me a call to arrange something.'

He showed me a series of modelling shots from his portfolio on his iPhone and it looked like he could take a picture. After months spent deliberately keeping myself off the radar, it felt strange to suddenly be noticed again, and for the right reasons. Ditto engaging in a social life once more, meeting up with friends I hadn't seen since before I got ill. I looked different but I felt like me again. There was colour in my cheeks and flesh on my bones. I felt healthy and vital.

Remembering to take my daily dose of tablets was my only concern and there were times when I'd get up in the middle of the night and pad downstairs to pop my forgotten Tamoxifen along with my aspirin, flaxseed oil, milk thistle and probiotic. But in the great scheme of things, how great that that was the only thing I had to worry about.

On the drive back home to the South of France after our six week road trip, we decided to break the journey and stop at a couple of hotels en route. I was swimming in a beautiful pool in the middle of the countryside in St Remy de Provence when it dawned on me that it was exactly a year to the day since I had found the lump that fateful morning in Florence. The previous 12 months had been a rollercoaster of emotions - fear, fury and hope, mainly - and swimming leisurely lengths in that peaceful pool with no other soul around was the perfect moment at which to realise that whatever else lie ahead, I had met this pisser of a challenge head on and not let it take me down.

One of the lasting legacies of treatment was that I lost a lot of deftness and turned into the clumsiest person on the planet. I've always been scatty, accidents seem to come and find me as you will already be aware. I can be swimming in the sea with a group of friends and the only jellyfish in the bay will somehow locate me and sting me three times while leaving everyone else alone.

The after effects of the drugs took my attraction to trouble to a new level. While the surf accident and the car crash were bad luck, falling backwards on the beach while putting up a parasol and crashing headlong into a rock the size of a Range Rover can only be described as freakishly bad luck. As I sat on the beach holding my dazed and bloodied head, a concerned holidaymaker ran over to help as the girls looked on worried and nauseous. 'Ça va?' he asked and I tried to nod as I touched the back of my head and felt the warm sticky patch of blood spreading across my hair.

I spent the next hour in the medical office being cleaned up yet again by yet more lifeguards, who were trying to persuade me to go to hospital for stitches.

'No more stitches,' I mumbled. 'I promise to sit quietly in the shade and not do anything hazardous.' I passed the rest of the day like an elderly lady taking in the sea air, sitting quietly and trying not to keep touching the red shock streak that had dried crustily at the back of my head.

'At least I have some hair to cover the lump,' I found myself thinking. 'It would have been a disaster if this had happened while I was still bald.'

My mammogram was booked for two days after my Piste to Plage ride on September 15th. Training rides on my newly repaired bike took my mind off this prospect. It was all about getting fit enough to ride, there was no room for any other concerns.

My first mountain training ride away from the flat coastal paths of Spain and Bordeaux involved a two hour climb into the Gorges du Loup near my home in 30 degrees of heat, and the sense of achievement I felt at reaching Gréolières, a tiny medieval village some 800 metres above sea level, was hard to explain.

I was proud of my body for hanging on in there throughout the grimmest of circumstances as the sweat poured off me and I cycled through tunnels, up gradients and round hairpin bends through spectacular mountain scenery. A piffling 20 km climb through the mountains on two wheels was nothing compared to walking 100 metres to the nurse's office in the village midway through chemo on legs that felt like they had been set in concrete.

And breathe…Make a daily To Do list and jot things down as they come into your head. Keep a notepad by your bed too. Without doing this, I would have struggled to remember pretty much everything.

Chapter Twenty Nine

One Year On

Writing this, one year on from discovering my lump, and casting my mind back to that time, it's painful to recall how crazy with fear I was. Trying to go through the motions every day, not betraying that anything was wrong to my children and keeping some kind of sanity in the three week limbo between tests and cancer diagnosis was one of the most difficult things I've ever had to do.

And then the real battle began, getting through the debilitating treatment, the months of fatigue, feeling dreadful and the inability to lead a normal life. You soon forget what normal feels like. But I made it, and if you find yourself in a similar position, just know this. You will be able to make it too.

As the first anniversary of being told I had cancer approached, I started getting nervy stomach cramps and sleeping very badly. The stress of my forthcoming scan, which was scheduled for the middle of September, weighed heavily on my mind. I seemed unable to focus or get anything done. My concentration was all over the place and instead of burying myself in work, which usually did the trick, I was drawn to the pool in the late summer sunshine with a book or some research to keep my mind from wandering. I felt in limbo, not unlike this time last year, except then I had a terrible sense of foreboding about the results of my biopsy, whereas this time I spent my days hoping and praying for a nice clean scan. The faintly queasy feeling of uncertainty didn't begin to compare to last year's sense of utter despair.

I also wondered whether my periods might be making a return as the pains were similar to the nasty premenstrual cramps I used to get. Then my imagination started working overtime and I found myself thinking: 'What if these pains mean it has moved to my ovaries? Or my liver?' The trouble with cancer, well, one of the many troubles with cancer, is that rational thought goes out the window and all sorts of irrational fears take hold. Although I'm not sure there is anything more nightmarish than waking up one day knowing that you are staring death in the face. As doom and gloom scenarios go, that one takes some beating.

Keeping going with the trivial stuff in life is the answer. With that in mind, I was tidying up Issy's room after she left for her first day back at school after the summer holidays and trying not to tut at the damp bath towels and dirty clothes all over the floor when I noticed a pin board that she had spent hours painstakingly decorating. Nestled in amongst the snapshots of our dogs Tallulah and Oscar and Issy and Liv fooling around with friends was a photograph of me relaxing with some friends on the beach during the holidays. What was telling about the inclusion of this picture was that it was me with a short peroxide crop. Not a picture Issy would have envisaged pinning up nine months earlier, given how distraught she was about my first and second short haircuts and the subsequent loss of my hair altogether. It proved how far we had all come on my rollercoaster of a journey and banished my annoyance at the damp towels and discarded clothing.

When she got home, I told her I was touched that she had included the photograph and she opened up about how hard she had found the previous year. 'When your hair started falling out, you looked really unwell,' she told me. 'I found that hard. I didn't like you putting on that freezing cold cap during your chemo either - I was scared about something so cold going on your head because you were so ill. But I knew you were going to be all right when your hair started growing back and you started looking normal again.'

My physical scars had faded to a fine line around the circumference of my right nipple and a small dent in the middle of my right armpit where my lymph nodes were removed. My right nipple had turned into a slightly lopsided flying saucer shape rather than the neat brown ring on the left. The worst scar, where my intravenous chemotherapy line was inserted, was a thick angry red line but nothing that a dab of concealer couldn't sort out. But the mental scars inflicted by the previous 12 months on the girls would take a lot longer to heal.

Liv told me: 'At the beginning, I tried not to talk to my friends at school about it because I hated the sympathy, and the comments of, 'Oh poor you, your mum has cancer.' If I talked about it, they would say they understood how I felt and I would think: 'No, you don't understand at all.' I would think about it when I was in the shower because I didn't have my iPad, computer or phone to take my mind off it. That's my thinking time, in the shower. And if I didn't talk about it, it was like it wasn't happening, I could zone out and that was easier for me.'

Issy agreed, adding: 'I didn't like talking about it either so I kept it to myself. I only told my closest friends and my teacher. If I didn't talk about it, I could pretend it wasn't happening. If anyone said how sorry they were, I would think depressing things and I wouldn't be able to get it out of my head.

'It frustrated me when people moaned about little things or said things like, 'Oh my God, I want to kill my mum, she is being so annoying.' I would have to walk away. Once, my best friend said something about her mum not allowing her out, and I had to say to her, 'If this ever happens to your mum, you won't even want to go out, you will just want to be with her.'

Liv told me that the hardest time was during my chemo. The girls would come home from school dreading how I might look. 'You were lying on the sofa, bald, really pale and sleeping and sometimes, it looked like you weren't breathing,' she revealed. 'That was the worst time for me. And I hated it when I found your hair in the bathroom sink. But the most worrying thing of all was that you seemed to always want to go out for lunch or do things with all of us together. That was when I thought, 'Oh my God, she wants to spend loads of time with us because she is going to die!'

Iain, who hates heart-to-heart chats like this, told me he coped by throwing himself into work and doing all he could to make life easier for me. A future without me weighed heavily on his mind. 'It was all about you getting better but I didn't always think you were going to get better,' he confided, his voice cracking with emotion. 'Sometimes I'd think, what if the worst happens, what do I need to prepare for? I wanted to make sure everything could run smoothly for the girls until they were ready to go off to university. I didn't really think about how it was affecting me, it was all about you and them. And much as it was hard to juggle everything, work really helped to take my mind off things.'

Random memories popped into my head. I remembered going for a swim in the sea 12 months earlier with Sarah while my girls stayed on the beach looking after her younger ones, organising sandcastle making competitions. I had to interrupt her bright chatter as we swam side by side around the bay to tell her I had found a lump. I remember reassuring her that everything would turn out okay as she struggled to swim, weeping and hyperventilating at the shock news of my dreadful discovery. I made her put a smile back on her face before we got out of the water to walk back up the beach to the kids like nothing was wrong. In summer 2012, on another beach in Western France, I reminded her of that conversation.

'You know when I told you everything would be okay and not to worry?' I said as she looked fearful. 'Well, I didn't say that because I thought it would be a false alarm. I knew it was going to be cancer, I don't know how I knew, but I just knew. I also knew that everything would turn out okay because it had to. There was no other possible outcome.'

'I knew that's what you meant,' she told me, her eyes filling with tears. 'And I knew it was going to be okay too.'

Summer 2012 turned out to be a blast. Getting out of bed and not being in pain, being able to walk to the bathroom rather than hobble and go out for a run or a punishing bike ride up the side of a mountain without feeling drained by the time I reached the top of the drive, were all things I no longer took for granted. Without a doubt exercise, the desire to be out in the fresh air and becoming more informed about my diet and what my body needed and, more importantly, what it didn't need, got me through as well as the unwavering support from my brave little gang of three.

And breathe…Think about incorporating supplements into your daily routine. A non-believer in supplements, I was swayed once I was diagnosed. As well as Tamoxifen, I take flaxseed oil, milk thistle, a 75mg aspirin and a probiotic every day. And I feel great.

Chapter Thirty

Rising To The Challenge

There's nothing like a goal to help you get through tough times and Piste to Plage was mine. Never mind that I signed up for it just days after embarking on a gruelling course of chemotherapy (or that I'd last ridden a bike rather badly 10 years earlier on a clubbing trip to Ibiza.) I'd read how Lance Armstrong kept going through his chemo with bike rides to remind him that he was still alive and it seemed to me that anything that could remind you of how good it feels to be alive had to be a positive thing.

The Help for Heroes fundraiser from the French ski resort of Sainte Foy to the Riviera was never going to be easy in weather that would range from driving rain and freakish September blizzards to 30 degrees of sunshine but boy, was it exciting.

It was a happy coincidence that the final day's ride fell the week before my first follow up scans and mammogram. While not taking away the anxiety and worry about what the tests would divulge, it did at least dilute my worries down to a manageable level.

As I lined up with 160 riders, including injured servicemen, in the pretty mountain village of Auron in early morning sunshine, the anticipation of the final descent from the mountains to the coast created a tangible buzz of excitement in the air. We pumped up tyres, slapped on sun cream and sat in the middle of the main street for a team photo and a final briefing on the day ahead.

At the forefront of my mind was the mantra 'DO NOT fall off the bike or the mountain.' Having fallen off twice on training rides, not falling off became an obsession, not least because a tumble at 50 km an hour would be likely to inflict more than a few cuts and bruises. I spotted crash barriers at the edge of a sheer drop that had already been crashed into and destroyed. Thankfully, it was nothing to do with me on this occasion.

We set off at 9.30am in staggered starts, with the slowest, most cautious riders first and the speed junkies last. I think you can guess which group I was in. The biggest group I'd ridden in before this was a petit gang of two so the joys of riding in a peloton were all new to me. The descent down from Auron through the mountain pass towards Nice is a spectacular drive at the best of times but on a bike with dozens of other riders whizzing alongside you, the wind on your face and the September sun high in a blue, blue sky, it came pretty damn close to perfection.

With the roads getting busier the closer we got to Nice, we bunched together with riders shouting out warnings about gravel, posts and oncoming cyclists to the riders behind. One minute you'd be on your own lost in thought or taking in the breathtaking scenery and the next, another rider would draw level and strike up conversation. I made a lot of new friends including Harry, an insurance boss from the UK, who appeared beside me on the approach into Nice.

'You're way too quiet, we'd better have a chat,' he said as I pedalled along the river path. 'How have you found the last three days then?'

'I'm only here for today and I love it,' I replied.

'Well you certainly chose the right day to join us but how come you didn't do all four days?'

When I explained that my doctors had advised against it following treatment, he nodded grimly.

'My wife had breast cancer,' he revealed. 'She is on her fourth year clear now. There's another guy riding with us whose wife had a double mastectomy. Are you on and off with the duvet each night too? That Tamoxifen plays havoc with your temperature gauge.'

He imparted the news that his wife's oncologist had advised her to continue on Tamoxifen beyond the recommended five year span, as it reduces the likelihood of a recurrence.

As we cycled towards the coast slightly ahead of schedule, the temptation to ditch the bikes for a dip in the sea proved too much and the grassy verge became a temporary bike park as 100 or so sweaty padded bottoms made a dash for a quick swim in the sea, much to the amusement of the French sun worshippers on the beach. 'Oui, c'est les Anglais,' sighed a female pedestrian as she looked on in bemusement.

If any of us needed reminding why we were taking part in such an arduous challenge, it came right then when Mark, a marine who lost his right leg below the knee in a parachute accident, abandoned his bike too, ran down the beach, kicked off his prosthetic limb and hopped into the sea amid deafening cheers. Jamie, a para who sustained 60% third degree burns when his plane cockpit burst into flames, Rab, an army captain who broke his back and neck in an army ski training session and Mike, an RAF operator injured during reconnaissance over Afghanistan, rode alongside us. However much your bum might hurt on that miniscule saddle, you wouldn't even contemplate moaning while riding alongside such inspirational human beings.

As we headed into the last few kilometres at Cap d'Antibes in a long meandering cycling snake, with drivers beeping and pedestrians cheering their support and shouting 'chapeau' at the sight of 160 riders in matching flouro coloured team shirts, the atmosphere was electric. We crossed the finish line in Juan-les-Pins to deafening claps and cheers from friends and family. There was no stopping the tears from flowing.

I didn't dare to dream that exactly a year after being diagnosed with cancer I would be marking that first anniversary riding in a challenge of this scale. It felt epic.

As the celebrations continued into the early hours at the after party on the beach in Juan-les-Pins, the buoyant mood made everyone dig deep at the auction and raffle. Altogether, we raised almost £400,000 for Help For Heroes to fund a hydrotherapy unit at Tedworth House rehabilitation unit in Wiltshire as well as spa facilities and a gym for injured servicemen.

Waking up the morning after the party, there was nothing to take my mind off my scans which were booked for the following day. In the weeks leading up to the scans, I had avoided making too many plans in case I received bad news. We had booked a trip to Florence months earlier to celebrate my birthday in October and while nothing was going to get in the way of that trip, I stopped short of planning a party or dinner with friends in case all was not well.

It's quite ridiculous to think that organising a curry night or a soirée with a few friends might jinx your recovery and mean a return of cancer because you dared to believe that you could plan ahead like a normal person but your mind goes into overdrive, analysing the tiniest irrational things that normal people wouldn't even notice.

Right up until the morning of my scan, I was getting twinges on the outer circumference of my right breast, which seemed to be saying, 'Presume nothing.'

I was in a pensive mood as Iain and I got in the car to drive to hospital. On the way there, we held hands as he rested one hand on the wheel.

'What if something's wrong?' I blurted out as we approached the hospital. I felt sick with fear.

'It's all going to be just fine,' he said but his eyes betrayed the fact that he was worried.

We sat in the waiting room, me armed with a year's worth of scans, reports and medical notes, him flicking through the headlines on the iPad.

'Madame Kershaw, s'il vous plaît.' The genial radiologist who had carried out my first mammogram one year earlier ushered me through to the little treatment room. He chattered brightly about how I should tell him if it was uncomfortable. Having a mammogram is a bit like being trapped in a lift door. The glass screen squashes your breast hard before photographing each aspect. It's uncomfortable, but not nearly as uncomfortable as the mental anguish of not knowing whether you have reason to worry.

'Ça va,' he trilled after photographing my left and right breasts. Did this mean everything was okay? I was led into another treatment room where the doctor who first diagnosed my lump was ready to carry out a further scan using a probe and gel.

'Le radio est normale,' he beamed. A big fat line had just been drawn under the worst year of my life. 'We just have to wait a few minutes for the results but don't worry, it looks like everything is fine.'

I walked back into the waiting room feeling like I could finally breathe out after a year of holding my breath in anticipation of the next twist or turn or piece of bad news. Iain glanced up, trying to anticipate my mood.

'He thinks it's fine,' I whispered as we squeezed each other's hands and I fought back tears of relief.

'Thank God,' he whispered back, struggling to control his bottom lip from quivering. 'I really don't want to cry in front of all these people.'

My year of living dangerously was officially over. And as you read this, I am still alive, still running, swimming, skiing, playing tennis and signing up for ridiculous challenges instead of putting my feet up with a glass of wine in front of the telly. Well, I do that sometimes too. Plus ça change.

And breathe....Keep a diary or blog to record how you are feeling and to look back on. That's how this book happened! Love and light to you all.

THE END

Some healthy recipes to get you started

Every morning, make your first drink a large mug of warm or hot water with half a freshly squeezed lemon and a dash of cayenne pepper at least 20 minutes before you eat breakfast. It cleanses your digestive system ready for the day ahead.

NUT BARS

80g flaked almonds

80g hazelnuts or pecans

80g walnuts

60g mixed linseeds and sesame seeds

100g dried cranberries

40g almond butter or peanut butter

125ml agave syrup

40ml melted organic coconut oil

¼ tsp salt

Put the nuts, nut butter and salt into a food processor and blend until coarse (not too smooth.) Add the agave syrup, cranberries and coconut oil and mix into a paste. Press down well into a small baking tray lined with greaseproof paper and chill in the fridge for an hour or two until hard. Cut into small squares or bars.

SPELT CHOCOLATE BROWNIES

200g white spelt flour

100g organic cocoa powder

1 ½ tablespoons baking powder

Pinch of salt

125ml organic vegetable oil

125ml agave syrup

125ml organic honey

125ml fresh espresso coffee

125ml organic milk

1 tablespoon vanilla extract

Grease and line a baking dish. Sift the flour, baking powder, cocoa powder and salt together in a large bowl. Mix the coffee, milk, vanilla, agave, honey and vegetable oil in a small bowl and fold into the dry ingredients, making a liquid batter. Pour into the baking tray and cook in a 170 degree centigrade oven for around 25 minutes. Check that the brownie is cooked with a skewer…it should be fudgy when you remove it. Allow to cool in the tray before cutting into squares.

SPELT LEMON LOAF

175g spelt flour

125g organic unsalted butter

2 large organic free range eggs

Zest of one lemon

125ml agave syrup

Pinch of salt

4 tablespoons organic milk

Juice of two lemons

100g xylitol

Grease and line a 450g loaf tin. Melt the butter and stir in the agave syrup, adding the eggs and lemon zest. Add the sifted flour and salt, folding into the wet ingredients and stir in the milk. Tip the batter into the loaf tin and bake in a 170 degree centigrade oven for around 40 - 45 minutes. If the top of the cake starts browning, lay a piece of greaseproof paper across the tin.

Put the lemon juice and xylitol in a saucepan and heat gently until the xylitol dissolves and the liquid becomes a syrup. When the cake is ready, pierce it several times with a skewer and pour the syrup over it while it rests in the tin. Allow to cool before removing from the tin.

Acknowledgements

This book is for all the women who assumed, like me, that life really does begin at 40 and refuse to even countenance the thought that it might be over before reaching 50. And for their long suffering partners, friends and family who might not realise what a key role they play in the battle.

I couldn't have written it without the support of the following people, who kept me going, made me laugh and gave me the strength, humour and faith to keep fighting even when I didn't much feel like it. Please forgive any omissions. You all know who you are in any case.

To my mum Carole, who became very au fait with her PC, sending me encouraging emails from London when she guessed I wouldn't feel much like talking, and who always told me not to answer if I didn't feel like it. To Justin and Lisa, Josh and Maddie, who never blinked when they saw the bald, fragile me. To Jean and Jim, my in-laws who despite their devastation never showed anything but support and Michael and Amanda, Gary and Phil and Claire and Brian, ditto.

To Sallyanne Sweeney, who saw something worth telling in my story and whose patience and attention to detail made it better than I could have hoped for and to Elle Macpherson, Simone Laubscher and my friend Amanda Holden for their kind words.

To Sarah, who always knew when to laugh or cry with me, Clare, who made me sea sick with her constant Skype calls, Sarah M and Angela, who recommended my fantastic nutritionist Simone, without whose highly effective food plan I could never have emerged from chemotherapy with energy levels that allowed me to lead a damn near normal life. To Sally for her quirky cancer care parcels which arrived just when I needed them. To Karin for her scissor skills and ability to say the right thing, Norma and Dr Sarah for their words of wisdom, Jackie for her cheering visits, Lissa in LA for her fajitas mix and Debi in Australia for her unwavering belief in my recovery. To Lisa V for herbal tea, dark chocolate, kind words and hand cream and Justin J for his highly entertaining home-made musical videos, they both showed discretion when I needed it most.

To my lovely, quirky, crazy friend Lisa H, whose own battle against cancer ended prematurely but whose laughter, battiness and thoughtfulness stay with me. And to Susie, Karen, Belinda, Mel and everyone else who kept in constant contact. Not one friend flaked out on me.

To my French crowd, Milly, who managed to make wig shopping a fun day out, Tony and Shan for countless hilarious lunches, Fi for making my cold hands warm again, Susie and Sylvia, who remembered every chemo session, Faye, whose yoga classes kept me buoyant and positive and Dawn, Graham, the two Helens, Neil, Harri, Abi and Christine, who showed unshakeable belief in me.

To my incredibly brilliant medical team, my GP Dr Ireland and doctors Lanvin, Largillier and Hoch at the Tzanck, who saved my life and showed kindness, care and attention to detail always. And to Sus, my wonderful, practical and kind nurse at the chemo unit, and her team.

Finally, to my husband Iain and our beautiful girls Liv and Issy. He made me laugh and was there with a squeeze of the hand, words of encouragement and compliments when I was at my lowest. He cooked supper, cleaned the house, rebuilt the pool and earned my living as well as his own. And to the girls, who tempered their concern, love and cups of tea with just the right amount of shirtiness, stroppiness and general teen dysfunction all designed to make me feel I'm not going anywhere just yet.

About the Author

Karen Hockney has 25 years of experience as a journalist, writing for UK newspapers and magazines on news, features, entertainment, travel, documentaries, film and music. She cut her teeth working with Piers Morgan at The Sun and her freelance clients include The Times, The Sunday Times, You Magazine, The Evening Standard, The Daily Mail, The Daily Telegraph, Heat and Hello. Karen lives with her husband and two daughters, dividing her time between London and the Côte d'Azur. She reports regularly from the Cannes Film Festival, the Monte Carlo TV Festival and MIPCOM.

Printed in Great Britain
by Amazon.co.uk, Ltd.,
Marston Gate.